Traditional Chinese Medicine

SHEILA MCNAMARA

& DR SONG XUAN KE

For Angela Palmer, my editor at the Observer magazine, the inspiration and guiding force behind this book

Copyright © Sheila McNamara and Dr Song Xuan Ke, 2012

The moral right of the authors has been asserted

All rights reserved. Without limiting the rights under copyright reserved above, no part of this publication may be reproduced, stored in or introduced into a retrieval system, or transmitted, in any form or by any means (electronic, mechanical, photocopying, recording or otherwise), without the prior written permission of both the copyright owner and the above publisher of this book

Contents

Acknowledgements 4

Introduction 5

Chapter One - Medicine on the Chinese Mainland 10

Chapter Two - TCM Ancient But Modern 20

Chapter Three - The Body as a Cosmos 29

Chapter Four - A Very Peculiar Practice? 39

Chapter Five - From the Casebook 52

Chapter Six - New Drugs from Old 74

Chapter Seven - Herbs and Their Uses 81

Chapter Eight - Eating for Health the Chinese Way 96

Chapter Nine - Qi Gong 106

Chapter Ten - Acupuncture 116

Chapter Eleven - Gynaecology 123

Chapter Twelve - In the Medicine Cabinet 127

Chapter Thirteen - A–Z 132

Appendix: The Ancient Manuscripts 194

Useful Addresses 204

Animal Products and Endangered Species 211

Bibliography 213

Index 214

Acknowledgements

There is a Chinese saying, 'A teacher even for one day is a parent for life'. In learning about traditional Chinese medicine (TCM), I have had several teachers, who in some instances have given not days, but weeks of their time to explain and elucidate the ways in which this ancient and impressive system of medicine works.

All are totally dedicated to their calling, and anxious that TCM should be more widely recognized and understood in the UK. All have patients who can, and do, testify to the effectiveness of TCM treatment in many kinds of disease. They share the hope – and belief – that by the twenty-first century, East and West will work together, incorporating their respective strengths to offer a more effective, less costly and readily available form of universal medicine that will be of benefit to all.

For their generosity, patience and kindness, I am indebted to:

- Dr Ruqui Chen, Chinese Medical Centre, Manvers Chambers, Bath.
- Dr Lorna Hsu, Pui-Yong Postgraduate School of Traditional Chinese Medicine, 53a Ormistone Grove, London W12 0JP.
- Dr Song Xuan Ke, Chinese Medical Clinic, Haverstock Hill, Hampstead, London NW6.
- Dr Bernard Lee, Fook Sang Acupuncture and Chinese Herbal Practitioners Association, 590 Wokingham Road, Earley, Reading, Berks RG6 2HN.
- Dr Shiming Lui (Associate Professor of Dermatology, Tianjin), Chinese Medical Centre, Manvers Chambers, Bath.
- Professor Kanwen Ma, Wellcome Research Institute, London.
- Dr Weize Wang (Associate Professor of Acupuncture, Tianjin), Chinese Medical Centre, Manvers Chambers, Bath.
- Acupuncturist Connie Dunne-Kirby, 20 Pearman Street, London SE1 7RB.

I am particularly indebted to Catherine Martin and Sino-European Clinics in Bath and in China for their help and kindness in all manner of ways, including allowing me repeated access to their medical centre, and to the doctors and staff of Tianjin First Teaching Hospital, and the Cancer Institute at the Academy for Medical Sciences in Beijing.

Thanks are also due to the many patients who so readily allowed me to sit in on consultations, read their medical records, and record their experiences of TCM treatment, in the hope that other people might derive the same benefit from the treatment as they themselves have done.

Introduction

Almost everyone in the UK has heard of traditional Chinese medicine. In recent years it has made the headlines many times. There have been stories of 'miracle' cures one week, and people being poisoned by unidentified remedies the next. This book sets out to avoid all the extremes and present a balanced picture.

My aim is to demystify the subject and give a general idea of how and why TCM works, and what its strengths and weaknesses are. TCM theory is totally different from orthodox medicine. Anyone who takes the trouble to read about it will discover a completely holistic system which acknowledges that mind and body are inseparable and exercise a profound influence over one another; that the malfunction of one organ will unbalance the rest; and that internal problems will have external symptoms, affecting the skin or the eyes, the mouth or the hearing. TCM treats the whole body, not just the illness.

The first question that readers probably want answered is, 'Can this type of treatment help *me*?' I hope they will find some guidance in these pages. A wide range of medical disorders is listed alphabetically in the A–Z (Chapter 13), making it easy for readers to use this for reference whenever the need arises. The information contained in the A–Z was compiled by Dr Song Xuan Ke, who studied from boyhood in his native China, and lectured at the College of Traditional Medicine at Canton before coming to practise medicine in Britain. This section explains in general terms what the TCM diagnosis is likely to be, and specifies the herbs likely to be used in the treatment. Readers can look up a particular complaint and read a generalized summary of its likely cause and treatment, before deciding whether they feel a course of treatment might be worth trying. One must always remember, however, that as TCM is a holistic system, no two cases are the same to a practitioner.

Many case histories are included, where patients talk about their personal experience of TCM. These were compiled over two years of research, the result of talking to patients who received treatment from many different doctors, and where possible, following their case histories. The experience of Western patients, most of whom seek help from a TCM doctor when all else fails, provides an especially useful guide for people who want to know more about how the system works before trying it themselves. Chapter 2 and the Appendix explain the history and development of TCM, and describe the work of the legendary doctors who advanced knowledge, conducted experiments and wrote the classical medical texts which are still in use today.

An outline of the medical theory is given, to explain to those who may be receiving treatment from a TCM doctor, precisely how the system works. It describes the marked differences in approach between allopathic and traditional Chinese medicine, showing how every organ in the body is affected by and in turn itself affects every other organ.

In TCM herbs are prescribed according to the anatomical channels on which they are said to act most effectively. Chapter 7 explains herbal lore and shows how herbs are classified, and the different ways in which they can be prepared.

The Chinese love to make their own medicinal broths and special dishes with ingredients which they believe will nourish and sustain them or help to cure illness. In Chapter 8 you can learn something of how foods are valued and how meals are balanced in China. All Chinese people are well versed in herbal lore, even if many of them are extremely sceptical about the old ways. Few of them, however, would deny the old saying that food was the first medicine, and most households in Hong Kong and mainland China will sit down to tangs (the Chinese word for soup), which have a medicinal purpose as well as being delicious to eat.

Perhaps the most mysterious aspect of TCM, like all things concerning the psyche and the subconscious mind, is qi gong. This is a system of mental and physical discipline which is the source of TCM. It involves breathing exercises which help to develop mind and body, so that people who study diligently can sense their own 'qi' (pronounced 'chee'), the energy force which flows through every living thing, and which practitioners believe can be harnessed to maintain good health or to hasten recovery from illness. This is the old tried and true philosophy of mind over the matter, given a special Chinese interpretation. Chapter 9 gives a resume of how it works. Readers who want to know more will find that this is a subject on which an increasing number of specialist books are being published.

Infertility is given a special place in the A–Z section, because as a journalist who has written many articles on the subject over a number of years, I know how widespread the problem is, and the sadness and misery it causes. TCM adopts a particular approach to this problem, and seems to be effective in treating cases where Western doctors can find no specific cause. The treatment is less intrusive and less drastic than in the West and does not involve the mental trauma that surrounds some forms of Western medical intervention such as IVF. It is also considerably less costly, though it may take up to a year of treatment, but in common with high-tech Western techniques, there is no guarantee of success.

Certain herbs used in TCM treatment of infertility are often extremely effective in increasing very low sperm count quite markedly. This is one area where the efficacy of the treatment can be speedily and conclusively assessed using modern scientific technology, and any childless couple where a low sperm count is a factor, might find a course of TCM treatment worth trying, particularly if clinical tests have already been conducted.

Acupuncture, the TCM therapy familiar to many people in the West long before they heard of Chinese herbal remedies, has been written about extensively. It is touched on briefly here (Chapter 10) because it is such an integral part of TCM that it cannot be ignored, but it is no more important, or more frequently used, than herbal treatments, which are less well known and less understood. Quite often doctors will practise both therapies. Readers who want to know more about acupuncture and moxibustion (which in its simplest form involves burning herbal cones on the needles used in acupuncture to reinforce the effect) can find many books which deal with the subject in greater detail.

There are now at least 600 TCM clinics scattered around the UK, and several colleges teaching TCM theory and practice to an increasing number of UK students. Chinese medicine is complementary in the very purest sense of the word. Its strengths lie in those areas where orthodox modern medicine is weakest. If it has sometimes been presented as a 'miracle cure', it is simply because it often succeeds where Western medicine has not yet found the answer.

There is nothing magical about TCM, however, and this cannot be emphasized too strongly. It has its failures, in precisely the same way as orthodox medicine does. Its medicines can also have side-effects unless prescribed by a qualified doctor. For example, there has been extensive debate in medical journals about patients who suffered from liver toxicity after taking herbs. Five fatalities have been recorded in Europe in recent years, some involving people drinking 'slimming' teas or taking other unprescribed herbs.

Compared with the tragic mishaps involved in synthetic drug therapy, however, these cases, sad as they are, are statistically insignificant. TCM doctors point out that their remedies are often thousands of years old, and have been tested throughout the generations from the time of recorded history. Mishaps can and do occur in all forms of medicine, because there will always be people who have rare allergies and experience unforeseen reactions, as in the cases of penicillin or certain types of anaesthetic.

In Europe today, thousands of patients have experienced TCM and have benefited greatly from it. They have found a cure for, or marked improvement in, diseases which they had previously been told were incurable. Chinese medicine does not cure multiple sclerosis, for example, but it does seem able to control the side-effects of that disease, – the blurred vision and incontinence, the relentless pain and the depression. Given immediately or soon after a stroke, acupuncture can hasten and enhance recovery, while arthritis, myco-enphalitis, menstrual disorders, skin problems, back pain and migraine, all seem to respond more favourably to the traditional Chinese approach.

The important thing to bear in mind when reading this book is that all the information it contains about diagnosis is necessarily very generalized. TCM is so very specific that it is quite impossible to give a completely accurate overall picture. Two patients with the same complaint will receive a totally different diagnosis, because the doctor's examination will reveal subtle differences in the symptoms. What the book provides is a reasonable guide to how TCM approaches each ailment listed.

The other point to keep in perspective is the way in which many Western doctors – perhaps the majority – reject TCM. With certain notable exceptions, they tend to be dismissive because TCM theory dates from pre-history, and uses archaic expressions such as wind evil penetrating the body or fire burning in the heart. This is simply because TCM, being as old as Chinese civilization itself, has never evolved a terminology of its own. Early Chinese doctors knew about the functioning of the endocrine system, the pituitary gland and the autonomic nervous system, but they described them in the lingua franca of the day, not in specially coined medical terms. Thus TCM does not express itself in the kind of professional terminology which can sometimes erect a barrier to understanding between doctor and patient in Western orthodox medicine.

Here in the UK, as the NHS dwindles to a mere shadow of its former self and people are increasingly required to seek private treatment for non-emergency conditions, TCM is destined to become much more popular and widespread. This brings us to the financial aspect. The legendary Yellow Emperor of China (see page 195) told doctors that they should spot disease in the early stages before it gained a hold on the body. Beginning treatment when disease was raging was, he said, 'like digging a well only when one feels thirsty. Is it not already too late?'

As previously mentioned, most patients in the West consult a TCM doctor when all else has failed. They are not so much thirsty as ravaged by drought, and the diseases from which they are suffering are usually chronic and require lengthy treatment. Although the fees charged by TCM practitioners are pretty much on a par with other forms of complementary medicine, and extremely modest compared with private Western medicine, they can sometimes put a strain on a limited family budget. All TCM doctors know of cases where patients responding well to treatment discontinue because of financial problems, or because the symptoms were cured, even though the doctor felt that the root had not been reached and the ailment might recur. Being aware of this problem, TCM doctors do what they can to help. Some have a reduced scale for pensioners or people on small incomes, and all will explain their scale of charges, and the expected length of treatment.

Some private insurance plans offer policies which will pay for TCM treatment. Many patients find they are able to discontinue modern drug treatment once they respond to TCM. In the future, perhaps patients who pay for TCM treatment will be able to reclaim a percentage of their previous NHS medication bill. With so much current emphasis on cost-cutting, and in a system where most general practitioners are fund-holders, an arrangement along these lines seems to be a fair and logical solution.

Some Western doctors offer acupuncture as part of their treatment, and more of them are now referring patients to TCM colleagues. Whether the two systems can or will ever be integrated is a matter for conjecture. What cannot be denied is that TCM, in Britain and elsewhere in the Western world, is here to stay. It has a significant contribution to make to the science of healing, and the West has much to learn from it.

CHAPTER ONE
Medicine on the Chinese Mainland

At six o'clock every weekday morning, a queue has already formed outside the main doors of the First Teaching Hospital of Traditional Chinese Medicine in the seaport city of Tianjin in Northern China. It stretches down the steps of the fourteen-storey building into the large forecourt with its central statue of a revered ancient acupuncturist.

Among the patients are squat Mongolians in Chairman Mao suits, with creased, leathery, smiling faces, tall Northern Chinese in anoraks and overcoats against the biting winter winds, bent old grandmothers, with short-cropped grey hair, in dark-coloured trousers and padded jackets, anxious mothers clutching the hands of wide-eyed children, and slender girls dressed in the latest Western fashions. The crowd is a microcosm of modern China, with its amazing blend of ancient and modern, just like the hospital which they attend.

The building, a square, grey, featureless concrete block, built in the 1950s, is just as lacking in aesthetic appeal as any of its Western counterparts of the same era. Inside are 800 beds, twenty medical and technical sections, and sixty-two outpatient departments. Yet the hospital is still hard-pressed to meet demand, and because the building cannot accommodate all the patients who need long-term nursing, special staff go out to care for a further 1,000 bed-patients in their homes.

When doctors at the hospital prescribe the old forms of treatment which have been tried and tested over thousands of years, they do so using a blend of Western and traditional diagnosis, aided by modern computer technology and bolstered by scientific research into the ancient remedies they prescribe. In the Intensive Coronary Care Unit, for example, a critically ill patient will be wired up to a monitor screen giving a constant reading of his heart action, in precisely the same way as an ICU patient in the West, but the drip in his arm highlights the difference between the two systems. The yellow liquid it holds is made from the gallstone of a bull.

This may sound more like the kind of concoction favoured by Macbeth's witches, but it works – so effectively, indeed, that one of the first skills a TCM doctor is taught is how to distinguish between bulls' and horses' gallstones. Only the occasional animal suffers from gallstones, and these are not discovered until after it is slaughtered. They are then extracted from the gallbladder, wound round with ricepaper pith, wrapped in writing paper made from bamboo, and hung to dry in a shady and draughty place.

The price for a bull's gallstone, which is much more efficacious, is scaled accordingly, and unscrupulous farmers often try to pass off horses' gallstones for bulls'. Why the gallstones of the bovine species should have greater curative qualities than the equine has not yet been established. What Western medicine does acknowledge is that bile from the gallbladder is a cholesterol-suppressant, so in the light of that fact, the treatment does not perhaps sound so outlandish after all. Gallstones are also used in treating fevers, stroke, infantile convulsions and epilepsy, and because they are comparatively rare, and so effective, they are a very expensive form of treatment.

In modern mainland China, there is little conflict between ancient and modern medicine, although there are of course plenty of young and Westernized people who pour scorn on the old treatments as a hangover from the dark ages, consider paracetamol far more acceptable than acupuncture for a headache, and could never be induced to swallow nasty-tasting herbs. In general, however, people know that both ancient and modern methods have their respective strengths and weaknesses.

Traditional Chinese medicine has had a chequered history in the course of this century. It fell into disrepute when the first Western doctors arrived in China, and attempts were made to ban it completely as 'unscientific' during the 1920s. This provoked a national outcry. The majority of people had great faith in the system, and were not prepared to see it disappear; the TCM doctors threatened an all-out strike. As a result, TCM continued unchallenged, and later, when Chairman Mao realized how vital it was to the health of the nation, he brought it back into favour and subsequently declared it one of China's 'national treasures'.

In China today, modern medicine continues to get the lion's share of the state's limited resources. None the less, TCM and allopathic practice co-exist in mutual harmony, balancing and complementing each other, in an ideal example of the first principle of Chinese medicine, the yin and the yang; the two opposing and mutually dependent sides of nature (see page 194). There are 450,000 doctors practising traditional medicine in China, slightly less than half the number who are trained in Western methods.

Government policy encourages co-operation between both types of medicine. If a patient develops an ailment which tends to respond quickly to herbal medicine, he will seek out a TCM doctor. If it is something which requires surgery, or an acute condition which Western medicine treats more effectively, he will opt for that.

As China currently changes over to a system of 'capitalism with a Chinese face', the system of medical provision is also under review. Health care for the entire population used to be free under the People's Republic. The money to pay for it came in part from central government who allocated a fixed amount per hospital bed, with the rest provided through the patient's work unit. Today, as in Britain, there is increasing emphasis on individual ability to pay.

Previously, in the case of non-working patients, 50 per cent of medical care was provided by the state, and the rest was donated from the work units of other relatives or – in rural areas – through the local collective. In urban areas work units continue to cover a large proportion of health care costs, but the current reforms and state funding shortages also mean that where possible people have to take responsibility for their own health.

Every city and town in China has at least one TCM hospital, and every village has its own TCM surgery. The country has over 2,000 TCM hospitals, thirty colleges teach TCM and 170 research institutes conduct modern high-tech studies into the therapeutic properties of Chinese herbs. The general view is that a system which has stood the test of time so convincingly is worth retaining, and if the instruments of twentieth-century science can help to shed light on how and why it works, so much the better. TCM, with 4,000 years of accumulated wisdom behind it, is still evolving, and is always willing to assimilate new scientific discoveries into its formidable body of empirical knowledge and research.

In a modernized Chinese city like Tianjin, with its population of 8 million, the largest Western medicine hospital is a streamlined, custom-built structure, with a helipad on the roof to fly in emergency cases, but at the other side of town, on Science and Technology Street, the TCM First Teaching Hospital is just as well regarded, and, in several departments, equally well equipped with the latest in modern medical technology.

As might be expected, it has a vast pharmacology section lined from wall to ceiling with archaic-looking medicine cabinets in which the thousands of herbs dispensed each day are stored. White-coated pharmacists scurry about between the aisles, carrying the old balances, which have a metal basket on one end of a weighted scale, as they add to the mounds of herbs they are heaping on to sheets of paper on the bench in front of them, which will be wrapped up and sent down to the dispensary for collection later.

In contrast, along the corridor, there are modern departments where diagnostic aids include a body scanner, an ECG machine and many other examples of sonic or electronic technology. There is a total of over 1,000 advanced medical instruments for clinical examination, diagnosis and treatment, including a computed skull tomography machine.

Because this is the teaching hospital attached to Tianjin's TCM College, it is constantly conducting studies into TCM management of disease, and claims some impressive results in the management of asthma, childhood epilepsy, coronary heart disease and diabetes. The hospital's paediatricians won a government award for their treatment of myocarditis in children, a viral condition in which the heart enlarges, causing extreme breathing difficulties and sudden death in critical cases.

One of the main herbs in their armoury against the disease is dansen (*radix salviae Miltiorizae*). Dansen, it has been proved, removes blood stasis and activates the blood circulation. At least twenty plants from the Materia Medica of China have this property. They are known in English as the ABC (activating blood circulation) drugs. According to the teachings of traditional Chinese medicine, blood stasis is a major factor in many diseases, and is detectable by a blue or purple tongue.

The children's cardiac ward was filled with young patients recovering from myocarditis, including a number of cases referred from other hospitals in the city. Their mothers help with the nursing, and stay in the hospital with their children, so stress on the little patient is relieved, and pressure on the staff reduced.

Western medicine remains relatively ineffective against viral infections like myocarditis, but TCM doctors use a variety of herbal combinations which can break down viral structures, something which Western medicine has consistently failed to achieve. In TCM terminology, the doctors are merely doing what their predecessors have done through the ages; perhaps treating a qi and yin deficiency, moving the blood, relieving heat and removing toxins, and clearing a heart obstruction. The language of diagnosis is unimportant; it is the results that count.

Unfortunately, Chinese research procedures do not always conform to stringent Western criteria and therefore tend to be discounted or ignored outside their own frontiers. Even when this is not the case, Chinese research papers are rarely published in other languages, limiting their accessibility for international scientists, who in many cases are very keen to get hold of them.

The Chinese Department of Health is now conducting a comparative study with other hospitals into the Tianjin myocarditis therapy, and the Japanese are doing their own research into some of the herbs used. No doubt some Western physicians will always look askance at the use of chopped earthworms or dried ge jie lizard (a type of gecko which looks like a small dragon), both of which feature in the TCM treatment of asthma, but it is increasingly likely that laboratory tests will reveal the active compounds they contain, and perhaps in the future they can be chemically reproduced for widespread application. In fact dried earthworm is now exported from China to the UK for use as medicine. It has a similar action to anti-histamine, and is very effective in easing respiratory conditions.

Most of the large Western drug companies are conducting research into the active compounds contained in Chinese herbs. While TCM practitioners are proud to demonstrate their skills and share their knowledge, the growing interest of the outside world in the secrets of the ancient Chinese remedies can present doctors with a dilemma.

For example, in the cardiac ward at Tianjin First Teaching Hospital, one very effective method involves an intravenous herbal medicine based on red sage and black aconite. ECG readings taken from patients who had suffered acute heart attacks thirty days previously showed the heart action to be almost back to normal after this treatment. Similar cases can take forty to fifty days when treated with Western drugs alone. When a patient is admitted complaining of acute pain, he is immediately prescribed a herbal remedy applied externally to the chest which is able to relieve the pain in less than twenty minutes. He is then given intravenous herbal medicines to tonify the qi and enliven the blood, plus acupuncture treatment to reinforce the body's defence system.

This particular formula has been devised by the head of the Cardiology Department, Dr Nu Yuan Qi, but it has not yet been given full trials in his homeland. If he were to allow the medicine to be clinically tested abroad with more readily available finance and facilities, it might be commercially developed there and the benefits lost to China. There are precedents for this. In the 1950s Chinese medical scientists were the first to develop insulin out of natural ingredients. They sent the formula to Hong Kong for production and it ended up being mass-produced in the colony and sold back to the Chinese as an imported product.

Chinese doctors are also confounded by the reluctance of the West to accept their findings because their methods of research do not readily conform to stringent Western standards. But even their strongest advocates admit that this is a serious flaw, and that exaggerated claims can be made for the efficacy of a treatment in the absence of thorough clinical tests. TCM relies too heavily on the experience of the practitioner, and is criticized, not unfairly, for sometimes lacking objective parameters.

TCM doctors respond to this by pointing out that double-blind tests cannot easily be conducted into some of their work. Moreover, the concept of giving one group of patients a placebo in place of the genuine article is ethically questionable to TCM doctors, for whom scientific detachment is secondary to the treatment of the sick. If a remedy is available to heal a patient, can a good physician be justified in giving a suffering person a bogus medicine, they ask.

Even when Western-style clinical testing is possible, and trials conducted to compare results between traditional methods and Western practice, the findings may be invalidated because some of the allopathic drugs used are Chinese copies of Russian drugs developed in the 1960s and 1970s, which have subsequently been either much refined or replaced by something more effective in the West. China is sadly behind the times in chemical drug therapy, lacking the financial resources to invest large sums in the latest pharmaceutical products.

Finally, there is the attitude of the Chinese public themselves. Like the rest of the human race when confronted with serious illness, they are prepared to try all forms of treatment in the search for a cure. But no matter how great their faith in modern medicine, in a crisis, old habits die hard. Every Chinese suburb will have some traditional healer or dispenser of folk remedies, with a local reputation as a medicine man. He may or may not be a qualified TCM practitioner, but his fame will be spread and enhanced by word of mouth, and the neighbourhood will have great faith in his abilities, when all else fails.

This presented real problems for specialists at the Cancer Institute at the Chinese Academy for Medical Sciences in Beijing, when they attempted to carry out a randomized study into a new form of treatment using both TCM and Western drugs. Because the study was long-term, it involved mainly outpatients, and it proved difficult to keep checks on how precisely they followed their prescribed treatment. Doctors discovered that a number of patients had also consulted the local medicine man and were taking his concoctions in addition to their hospital drugs.

Despite such minor setbacks, however, medical and scientific institutes throughout the world are now beginning to look with great interest at the work done in TCM hospitals, and many – particularly in the UK, Japan, Germany and the United States – are conducting their own clinical trials into herbal remedies. It is widely recognized that several herbs long used in TCM have the ability to bolster the body's own immune system to enable it to fight diseases like cancer, and even AIDS, and that a number of herbs can lessen the side-effects of chemotherapy and radiotherapy, reducing sickness and enabling the patient to cope with the stress of treatment. In skilled hands, acupuncture can do the same.

In 1975, physicians from several hospitals and medical schools throughout China organized a fu-zheng therapy co-ordinating group to study the efficacy of several traditional herbs as biological response-modifiers in cancer patients. Fu-zheng, which literally means promoting or enhancing the body's own defence mechanism, is the first principle of TCM treatment. Patients with different types of cancer at various stages were put on a two-month course of fu-zheng medicine to augment their Western treatment, and results showed that the side-effects were significantly reduced.

From that initial research, further work was carried out in the mid-1980s on herbs such as *Astragalus membranaceus* and *Ligustrum lucidum*, both of which were shown to have properties which helped to bolster the patient's defence mechanism, protect the bone marrow, liver and adrenal cortical function, and decrease the incidence of gastric toxicity. Subsequent studies in China and in the Department of Clinical Immunology and Biological Therapy in the University of Texas Cancer Center showed that extracts from several traditional herbs could reactivate the immune system to a greater or lesser degree. *Astragalus membranaceus* in particular could completely restore a failing immune system and return its T-cell function to normal.

Now that China has an open-door policy, many doctors in the West are eager to learn more about these treatments, and there is a great sense of national pride that TCM is at last attracting recognition and respect abroad. Outside interest, including the increasing number of students from abroad studying at Chinese medical colleges, provides finance to equip the wards better and to fund further research.

All the major colleges and hospitals in China are encouraging foreign students to enrol for study courses and seminars, and, in common with hospitals in the West, each is likely to have its specialist areas of excellence. Tianjin's TCM College is a clinical research centre for acupuncture and moxibustion, teaching foreign students from all over the world. It also has several distinguished doctors practising in the UK, at clinics in Bath and

Manchester, in a joint Sino-British operation which, in its own small way, points to a future in which medical exchanges will become more widely accepted.

In their native China, all the doctors participating have consultant status, have trained in Western medicine as well as TCM, and are highly motivated to respond to any approaches from UK hospitals which might be interested in learning at first hand about their work. Slowly, progress is being made. A hospital in Bristol is to conduct a study into the response of patients taking TCM for a variety of skin complaints, with the blessing of the local health authority. The Royal Free Hospital in London is planning to recruit a Chinese dermatologist to help with its research.

The president of the Tianjin hospital, Professor Shi Xuemin, is an expert in China on acupuncture, in particular as a post-stroke therapy. He has devised a treatment called 'xing nao kai qiao' (meaning 'to wake up the brains and open the mind') which is widely used at home and abroad. Patients from Western hospitals in the city are sent over for rehabilitation. Surprisingly, although acupuncture is respected and readily available in Britain, it does not seem to have much of a history in post-stroke treatment here. This is regrettable, since in many cases it has a beneficial effect in restoring mobility, and the earlier it is given, the faster and more effective the response.

Professor Shi has also developed a cerebral thrombosis capsule, made from a herbal prescription which is produced at the hospital's own pharmaceutical factory and has been patented for general sale. Several of the leading consultants have similarly produced their own patent medicines. After submitting their prescriptions of herbal remedies to government scrutiny, they apply for patents to produce the medicines commercially. Trials are first conducted on selected patients and then submitted to the TCM Management Bureau, which collates all the data on prescriptions and scrutinizes the results of clinical and laboratory trials on efficacy, toxicity, etc. If approval is given, the prescription is passed on to a pharmaceutical manufacturer for commercial production, and is sold all over the country, as well as from the little stall on the ground floor of the hospital.

Patent medicines are just as popular in China as they are elsewhere in the world. Everyone buys over-the-counter preparations for minor ailments, or to try to hasten recovery in more serious cases, and many brand-names are as famous and as highly regarded as Western ready-made remedies for colds and flu or arthritis pains. Some date back thousands of years, and were first recorded in some of the ancient classics, a fact that Chinese doctors often emphasize when answering criticism about the lack of scientific research into drug treatments in China.

TCM can also claim some special success in treating cases of epilepsy. In Tianjin First Teaching Hospital, a fairly typical case was that of a teenage girl who became epileptic after an accident seven years previously. She was responding to herbal medicine and acupuncture, and had been entirely free from attacks for a month. The case was referred by in Tianjin's Western hospital where they were unable to prevent the severe fits she had been suffering at ten-day intervals.

Another teenager, an epileptic for eight years, was sent over by colleagues in the Western hospital, when her condition worsened to the point where she was having sixteen fits a day. After four weeks on a regime of herbal medicine and acupuncture, the condition was controlled to one fit a week. Patients in Britain can also testify that epileptics respond well to TCM treatment (see page 56), although doctors emphasize that it is a difficult condition to cure, particularly when long-established, and sadly nothing can be done to repair the neurological damage which occurs in severe cases.

The particular epilepsy treatment developed at Tianjin is being clinically tested in a Beijing hospital under the auspices of the Department of Health, and the doctors were invited to present a paper on their work at an International Conference on Epilepsy in Barcelona. Unfortunately they were unable to attend because of lack of finance – a common problem in emergent China, and another hurdle along the road of East–West medical co-operation.

Many of the wards in Tianjin's First Teaching Hospital contain patients who have failed to respond to modern medicine, although it has to be borne in mind that as previously mentioned 'modern' can sometimes refer to drugs discontinued or replaced in the West a decade or so ago. However, although it is hazardous to make comparisons with the kind of drug therapy sufferers would receive in a hospital in the UK, this does not devalue the results achieved by the TCM doctors. The wards at Tianjin are full of cases which would challenge consultants in the developed world. A thirty-year-old patient who had been diagnosed as schizophrenic at the city's Western hospital the previous year was transferred to the TCM hospital when he failed to respond to orthodox treatment. Here doctors diagnosed his complaint as insomnia and restlessness, two of the main symptoms of his condition, and treated him with acupuncture. After several months, he had recovered sufficiently to be allowed home, and though continuing as an outpatient, was able to return to work.

TCM always looks first for the root cause of any physical disease, believing that once this is treated, the symptoms will clear up automatically. The principle of treatment in mental illness is to calm and settle the shen – the spirit – which, not unlike the Western concept, is part-emotion, part-mind. It is believed to reside in the brain during the day, and to rest in the heart at night. If it is disturbed, irrational behaviour and sleeplessness automatically follow. Treatment to calm and settle the shen will concentrate on the liver as well as the heart. Neither is an organ that modern anatomy associates with mental disorders.

Although things are changing so rapidly in China that it is difficult to keep pace with progress, it is still an emerging country, with a long road to travel towards modernity and prosperity. Hospitals are not as streamlined or as clean as in the West. It is not unusual for an emergency patient to arrive in Casualty pushed by relatives on a handcart, but once admitted, patients will be treated with the same skill, dedication and expertise as in any modern and sophisticated hospital in the developed world.

In the Casualty Department, only the most experienced doctors are in attendance. Unlike in British hospitals, where newly qualified young housemen tend to cut their medical teeth in the Accident and Emergency Department before going on to the wards, the learning skills of TCM doctors are acquired on the wards, where new doctors spend a lot of time gaining experience before they are considered to have the necessary expertise to diagnose in Casualty.

In a small, cramped and crowded Casualty Ward in Tianjin, four doctors typically handle seventy patients each in a three-hour morning surgery, diagnosing by traditional methods which include reading the pulse and examining the tongue. Russian lecturers from the Pavlov Institute in St Petersburg, on a three-month study course in winter 1993, declared themselves astounded at the speed and accuracy with which the Casualty doctors worked. In weeks of working alongside them, they said, they had yet to encounter a case where a doctor had given a faulty diagnosis.

Research has also started at Tianjin First Teaching Hospital into a new approach to diabetes. A husband-and-wife team are investigating a treatment which appears to restore the B cells which manufacture insulin in the body. In a country in which 1.2 per cent of the population (20 million people) are diabetic, the prospect of a breakthrough in this field would have profound implications. Patients on 300-mg insulin injections per day were able to have their dosage reduced to 200 mg, and sugar levels in acute cases can be restored to normal in ten days.

Even in a hospital as forward-looking as the one at Tianjin, the old ways are not neglected: in the large physiotherapy gym, a corner is set aside for qi gong practitioners, who treat their patients with a strange series of hand passes over their bodies.

Qi gong is basically a method of meditational exercise involved in the cultivation of physical and spiritual perfection. It is considered the forerunner of TCM, since qi, the 'subtle breath' or the 'life energy', is at the heart of everything and the very wellspring of human existence. Gong is another word which defies literal translation. It means something between 'cultivation' or 'achievement' and implies that with long practice, the qi can be harnessed and controlled to maintain health, serenity and vigour, and to help ward off illness.

All TCM doctors are taught qi gong, and some specialize in using it as a treatment. They work by transferring their own qi to the sufferer, and claim to know exactly where the patient's energy channels are blocked or are at their weakest. The very highest Grand Masters of qi gong are said to develop such sensitivity to their patients that they 'see' the blockage merely by looking at the patient. For more about qi gong, see Chapter 9.

Although some TCM doctors are sceptical about the efficacy of qi gong as a treatment, none have reservations about the discipline, which was developed during the Han Dynasty and is at its most useful when privately practised as a system for promoting good health, rather like yoga, or its own derivative, tai qi. Qi gong remains at the very root of TCM, and at their daily healing sessions the qi gong masters certainly seem to bring pain-relief and improvement to their patients. This may owe something to the placebo effect, but it would be wrong to dismiss it out of hand. Until very recently, Chinese herbal medicine itself was regarded by Westerners as primitive and largely ineffective. Just how prejudiced and misguided that view was, we are only now discovering.

CHAPTER TWO
TCM Ancient But Modern

The work of dedicated medical men, absorbed in their own research, meticulously recording their clinical observations and scientific study, has expanded the knowledge of TCM practitioners throughout the millennia, right up until the present day, when it is once more being recognized as a science with much to offer the outside world. TCM is far from being a fossilized system, rooted in the dark ages. It has evolved, one step at a time, over the centuries. It is still evolving today.

Bian Que, also known as Ch'in Yueh-jen, probably lived in the second century BC. He had great gifts as a diagnostician and went out of his way to demystify medical practice. The achievements of this legendary medical man were recorded in the Imperial Annals of the Han Dynasty. He is said to have carried out a heart-swap operation between two patients whose illnesses stemmed from opposing malfunctions of that organ. If all the exploits attributed to him are true, he must have been around for 400 years, and travelled the length and breadth of China. In fact it is thought that the name may actually have been a respectful title applied to gifted doctors over the course of four centuries, and the experiences of a number of them may have been erroneously attributed to one man. He made a major contribution to traditional Chinese medicine, and a number of stories illustrate this.

In one, the son of the King of Guo lay dying, and the court physicians could do nothing to help. There was just one doctor in the whole of China whose skills might save the boy, if only he could be brought there in time.

Bian Que was duly summoned, and arrived at the royal palace to find the court in mourning. The crown prince was being prepared for burial. 'My son might have been alive if you had come sooner,' lamented the king, but the sage asked to be shown the body. His examination confirmed his suspicion that the prince had actually lapsed into a deep coma. He immediately gave acupuncture treatment to revive him, then applied compresses soaked in a decoction of herbs.

Within hours of his arrival, the patient was able to get to his feet. The doctor then prescribed medicines which restored him to full health in twenty days. Unsurprisingly, outside the gates of the court among the common people, rumours spread that here was a miracle-worker who could raise people from the dead. Pien Ch'iao assured them: 'I cannot bring the dead back to life. The prince still had some life left in him. I simply found the spark and fanned it into a flame.'

Whatever the true identity of Bian Que, his legend survived, and so did the legacy he left to his profession. He laid down the classic diagnostic rules which practitioners still follow today.

Bian Que gave six reasons for serious sickness:

- Living a life of dissipation.
- Putting the love of money above health.
- Poverty; eating the wrong food and wearing inappropriate clothing.
- An imbalance in the yin and yang energy in the body.
- Being too emaciated to swallow medicine.
- Believing in sorcery instead of doctors.

Bian Que was the first exponent of pulse-reading, and devised the TCM procedure of the Four Examinations. He advised listening carefully to the sounds the patient made and asking for details about the course of the disease and its symptoms. He taught that every illness leaves its own hallmark on the surface of the body, and that all sickness gives many outward signs that the diligent physician should be able to recognize.

To this day, TCM continues to follow the procedure that Bian Que advocated:

- Doctors still look first for the outward and visible signs of disease.
- They follow a rational and empirical science which has no connection with mystery or magic.
- They continue to follow the theory that diseases start superficially and penetrate deeper into the body as they advance.
- Every disease is diagnosed by the Four Examinations.
- Pulse-reading is generally regarded as perhaps the most important diagnostic tool of all.
- They still treat around 300 conditions with acupuncture and moxibustion and, incidentally, still use a point on the upper lip, directly beneath the nose, to restore patients to consciousness.
- The herbal decoctions they prescribe today have remained largely unchanged for hundreds of years.

Bian Que developed his theories out of the solid framework of the *Nei Jing*, the celebrated *Yellow Emperor's Classic of Internal Medicine*, which is the oldest and most revered of the 8,000 medical books in China's national treasury. It teaches the three basic tenets in which all TCM theory has since been rooted: the Tao, the natural law which includes the human body as a mirror image of the cosmos; yin and yang, the mutually dependent opposites, of which all things created are either one or the other; and the five elements, or the five transformation phases, which represent the eternal circle of growth, vigour and decline.

Bian Que's own book, the *Nan Jing*, or the *Difficult Classic*, which interpreted and explained the more complex parts of the *Nei Jing*, has become a valued classic in its own right. All the famous Chinese medical sages did precisely the same. They advanced medical knowledge through their own clinical practice and observations. They researched and analysed the teaching of previous classics, revised and updated them in the light of the latest findings. In this way, medical theory was expanded to include the eight principle syndromes to which all diseases belong: yin and yang, interior and exterior, cold and heat, deficiency and excess.

The eight principles enabled doctors to identify illness not just by the organ at the root of the problem, but by four further classifications. If, for example, the patient is suffering from flu, with a stuffed-up nose, sore throat and severe headache, the doctor will classify his condition as an external condition, because it is not rooted in the internal organs. If other symptoms such as fever, dry mouth or thirst are present, this will suggest too much heat. So overall this condition is classified as an external syndrome, of excessive heat. As all these are yang characteristics, this would be a yang disease.

In the Qing Dynasty (1644–1912) Ye Tian Si developed Bian Que's powers of medical detection into the theory of the Four Levels, which described with clinical precision the progress of diseases such as meningitis. The theory has since become an integral part of TCM diagnosis.

Ye taught that there were four stages of heat in diseases marked by fever:

Wei: An exterior syndrome, indicating the superficial invasion of the body, affecting the defensive energy, and characterized by feverishness, headache, thirst, cough and sore throat.
Qi: In which the heat enters the blood, causing sweating and high temperature, thirst and a rapid pulse.
Ying: Which indicates a serious invasion of the internal organs, indicated by delirium, and 'tide' fever in the afternoon.
Xue: A critical stage at which the blood vessels are damaged, and the patient may begin to bleed through the skin and lapse into coma.

Today, in research institutes all over China, scientific studies are being conducted into pulse-reading, tongue diagnosis, acupuncture and ancient exercises for physical and spiritual development. Many of the findings confirm what the sages taught centuries ago. In China efforts continue to integrate the traditional system with modern Western medicine, and TCM is adjusting its boundaries once more to encompass the body of biochemical knowledge which has advanced so rapidly this century.

Although a combined system works well in China, the chasm between Eastern and Western medicine can sometimes appear insurmountable. Modern science expects proof, TCM relies on results – hence the difficulty Western medicine finds itself faced with regarding the practice of acupuncture, for example.

That acupuncture has a therapeutic effect is no longer disputed. There is substantial evidence to show that it stimulates endorphins in the brain, which produce clinical analgesia. How and why are different questions. No one knows how the channels through which the qi, or life force, travels were discovered. They are entirely separate from the circulatory or nervous systems, or any other concept of modern physiology. Unlike the blood vessels, some of which can be glimpsed with the naked eye under the surface of the skin, the network along which the qi flows cannot be seen, although its existence has been established by modern researchers tracing the flow of energy with semiconductor diodes.

Many Western doctors continue to insist that since dissection cannot reveal the channels, or meridians, they cannot be accepted as anatomical facts. They are no more than a quaint and fanciful attempt of early man to explain the functions of the human body. By way of contrast, when in nineteenth-century Britain the distinguished Scottish scientist James Clerk Maxwell established the existence of radio waves by pure equation, he was able to demonstrate his theory by means of equipment which harnessed the waves.

The equipment which demonstrates the existence of the energy channels of acupuncture is the human body itself. When pain is relieved or illness cured by tuning into it at particular points with a set of needles far from the site of the disease, that still does not constitute proof as far as rational science is concerned. Relief or cure continues to be interpreted as the possible result of a mega placebo effect. Taking that argument to its furthest conclusion, we might wonder if it is all in the mind when we tune in to the shipping forecast on Radio 4.

Theories abound about the discovery of acupuncture. One holds that it happened in the Stone Age when men using tools made from sharpened stones observed that if they accidentally punctured one part of the body, a pain or a problem often cleared up in another location. Another claims that it was first observed by soldiers, wounded by arrows, who noticed that other ailments they suffered from seemed to disappear afterwards. The most popular and most likely belief is that the ancient doctors gradually discovered the channels through observing the tender spots on a patient's body as they carried out examinations.

Many of the acupoints do indeed announce themselves by their sensitivity. It is also quite common for some patients to feel the sensation not just in the area around the needle, but along the whole length of the particular channel. The pain of angina, for example, is frequently experienced from the chest and down the arm, precisely the pathway of the heart channel which runs from the heart to the little finger.

Acupuncture has been in common use since the dawn of civilization. Oracle bones dating from the twenty-first century bc show that it was practised in those times using stone slivers called bian. By the eighth century, metal needles had been introduced and gold acupuncture pins were recently excavated in Hubei province in a tomb dated at the third century BC.

It is important to stress that needling, as it is often called, is only one therapy in classical medicine, and not the most widely used. It has a strong association with TCM in the Western mind primarily because it is so different from any therapy practised in the West, and because it has had more publicity. It made headline news all over the world during Richard Nixon's state visit to China in 1972, when one of the pressmen covering the trip developed appendicitis. James Reston, a columnist for the *New York Times*, wrote an account of his appendectomy, performed under acupuncture and local anaesthetic, describing how he remained conscious throughout. After surgery, more acupuncture and moxibustion were given to hasten the recovery, and Reston reported that 'the swelling went down within an hour and the pain never came back'.

His report went around the globe. Newsreel films showed patients having all manner of major surgical techniques carried out in Chinese hospitals while they remained fully conscious, getting off the table and walking back to the ward afterwards. It seemed miraculous, and to some extent, it was. But the use of acupuncture in surgical operations is not as widespread as is sometimes reported, and would not work in all cases. Bian Que and another ancient practitioner, Hua Tuo, both used anaesthetics which they had developed themselves. The formula has been lost in each case, but possibly contained cannabis or opium. Both men were extremely skilled in needling, as the stories told about them illustrate, and presumably they would have used acupuncture to sedate their patients if it had been entirely effective for that purpose.

Today, in Chinese hospitals combining modern medicine and TCM, acuanalgesia, as it is called, may be used in abdominal surgery. It can greatly assist post-operative recovery, and there will be no need for the patient to fast beforehand. It may also be used on patients with heart conditions where a general anaesthetic might prove hazardous. It is not, however, part of the cultural tradition, and was introduced after 1958, the year in which Chairman Mao declared that modern medicine and traditional medicine should 'serve the people side by side'.

James Reston's experience was far from the first time TCM had commanded attention in the West. Europe got its original insight into traditional Chinese medicine in the fifteenth century, when it was reported by the Jesuit missionaries. The eminent English physician Sir John Floyer (1649–1734) was so inspired by a translation of an ancient book on the art of feeling the pulse that he devised a pulse watch, the earliest of its kind.

Some Chinese herbs, such as smilax China-root, came into vogue in sixteenth-century Europe. The Chinese method of inoculation against smallpox was introduced into England in the early eighteenth century. Smallpox was not a disease native to China, and is thought to have been brought into the country by traders using the Silk Road. In the Sung Dynasty (AD 960–1279), a famous general called Ma Yuan and many of the soldiers in his army died during a smallpox epidemic. Later, the son of the prime minister developed the disease, and a philosopher living in the O Mei mountains at Szechuen was reputed to have inoculated the child.

A classic entitled *The Golden Mirror of Medicine* gave the formula for the inoculation of children in 1713. Powdered smallpox scabs were to be laid on cotton wool and placed in the nostrils which were then plugged for several days. Twenty scabs were used for a year-old baby, thirty for an older child. The procedure by no means guaranteed success. Some children actually died, though many more were saved. Later, the internationally famous scientist Li Shi-zhen recorded using cow fleas to inoculate against smallpox, predating Edward Jenner's work in the West by 100 years.

The toll taken on children by constant smallpox epidemics led to the development of paediatrics in China, and the inoculation process employed against the disease was one of the things that impressed the Jesuits, who wrote in some detail about Chinese medical practices. The Jesuit d'Entrecolles observed that, 'If the powder is inserted in the nose and a fever breaks out, if the pustules do not appear until the 3rd day it is guaranteed that out of 10 children, 8 or 9 will be saved. If the pustules appear on the 2nd day, 5 out of 10 will be at considerable risk. Finally, if the pustules appear on the first day, not one of the 10 children will be saved.'

The Jesuits had the same reaction to TCM as many people have today. Father Dominique Parrenin, who died in 1741, confessed, 'When I hear Chinese physicians speak on the principles of illness, I do not detect any accuracy or veracity in their arguments, but when they apply to their patients remedies they have devised through taking the pulse and examining different parts of the head, I see that such remedies practically always have a beneficial effect.'

The problem faced by Chinese medicine was that charlatans flourished alongside genuine physicians, and always had done. The fortunes and development of the profession were always very much affected by historical events. China's turbulent history of a seemingly endless cycle of warfare, invasion, tyrannical rule and Golden Ages, ensured that in one era medicine would be termed 'the benificent art' and physicians revered as 'the hand of the nation', while in the next, it would be totally discounted or doctors subjected to persecution.

By the time the Jesuit Matteo Ricci arrived in China from Macao in 1582, there were no laws preventing anyone from setting up in medical practice. Matteo noted this fact in reports home, and condemned 'the stupidity of alchemy and the sellers of immortality'. The presence of these cranks and quacks often brought genuine medicine into disrepute.

Despite the fact that the early medical books were revered among literary men and philosophers alike as the very best of the nation's classics, and there had been medical state examinations from the tenth century BC, the profession was not always held in similar esteem. Confucius decreed that doctors were not gentlemen and scholars, but artisans, and it was not until the Sung Dynasty (AD 960–1279) that the Imperial Bureau for Medicine was established and an Academy for Medicine opened in Beijing, mainly to minister to the Emperor. Students were expected to possess a thorough grounding in all the medical classics and the examination system ensured that only the most proficient got through.

In 1027, the Emperor Wang Anshi had two life-size copper anatomical figures made which contained all the channels and had holes pierced to mark all the acupoints. At the examinations, the hollow statues were filled with water, and a coating of beeswax completely hid the holes from view. The students had to demonstrate their needling prowess by hitting the right spot each time. If they were successful, water poured from the hole.

The Sung Dynasty was a settled and prosperous time which saw the beginning of many of the scientific advances for which China became famous. Forensic medicine was encouraged, and autopsies carried out on executed prisoners. Woodblock printing and the invention of moveable type meant that books were widely available. Anatomical plates were introduced to show the organs of the body, and doctors were instructed in physiology, histology and various other disciplines involved in the practice of medicine.

Prosperity declined again as the ages passed, and war, famine, pestilence and death were familiar visitors to the Chinese. As long ago as the Han Dynasty, Zhang Zhong-Zhing had recorded that two-thirds of the people in his native village died of disease in a ten-year period, 70 per cent of them from typhoid. By the time of the Western missionaries in the sixteenth century, epidemics of bubonic plague, cholera, dysentery and parasitic diseases were commonplace; and when the Great Powers arrived to manipulate the ailing Qing Dynasty, signing treaties in 1824, hospitals dispensing Western medicine began to be set up, offering a completely new and very successful form of treatment to those who had access to it.

The mass of the people, still living feudal lives far distant from the sophistication of China's capital or major trading cities, continued to rely on local doctors and folk medicine. Foreign observers often could not (or did not take the trouble) to distinguish the good from the bad, or the quack from the genuine traditional doctor. It all sounded like mumbo-jumbo to them, and before long many of the educated Chinese were thinking the same way. It was only a matter of time before Chinese students started going abroad to learn Western medicine. The first of them, a doctor named Huang Kuan (1828–79), left Canton to study at Edinburgh University.

When the nationalists took over in 1911, modern China came into being, founded by a man who had himself qualified in Western medicine in Hong Kong. Dr Sun Yat Sen's aim was the modernization of the country. 'If we do not learn what has been done better abroad, we will sink into backwardness,' he told the people. His Minister of Education urged the banning of traditional medicine, and in 1929 an edict forbade the opening of new schools teaching old-style medicine, while doctors who continued in practice were strictly controlled. Censorship ensured that no more papers on advances in traditional medicine could be printed, to halt the spread of 'unscientific information'.

The move aroused fierce protest, and angry supporters of traditional medicine met in Shanghai and formed the National Association for Chinese Medicine. Although the government attempted to ignore this, and continued on its path towards medical 'progress', it eventually had to concede defeat. A treatise published by the World Health Organization in 1983 explained why.

People continued to believe in it. It cured illness that Western medicine apparently could not cure. Medicinal plants were widely available, relatively inexpensive, practical, easy to use and had few adverse effects. Thirdly, it was based on an unique theoretical system, notably with regard to the concepts of yin and yang, vital energy and of blood, that modern medicine could neither replace nor explain.

Furthermore, there was the same diversity in the quality of those practising Western medicine as there was among herbal doctors. A report in 1943 stated that only 60 per cent of them were properly qualified. There were, in any event, nothing like enough allopathic practitioners to attend to the needs of the most highly populated country on earth, so if TCM had been outlawed completely, the mass of the people would have been left without any medical help at all.

In the 1930s Mao Zedong placed health care high on the list of priorities but the task facing him was daunting. By 1949, estimates put the ratio at one doctor for every 1,100 of the population. At the first National Conference of the People's Republic in August 1950, Chairman Mao made the call that changed the face of medicine on the Chinese mainland: 'Unite, all medical workers, young and old, of the traditional school and the Western school, and organize a solid front

There were no figures then to show precisely how many doctors the country actually had, but six years later it was estimated that there were 500,000 traditional physicians and 12,000 practitioners of Western medicine. Health centres were set up in every district, and new standards of hygiene were encouraged. Between 1950 and 1965, cholera, plague, smallpox, opium addiction and many nutritional diseases were almost eliminated, and by 1966 thousands of health auxiliaries were trained – nurses, midwives, laboratory technicians, and the famous 'barefoot doctors'. These were ordinary workers given a grounding in basic medical care, so that they could bring reasonable standards of treatment and health care to the countryside. In fact they were never barefoot. Their name was derived from a translation of the Chinese word which actually means agricultural worker, because work in the paddy-fields was done barefoot.

In 1971, society was 'remoulded' and hygiene was regarded as honourable. The Great Patriotic Health Movement was set up to eliminate 'the four pests' and people had to spend their spare time killing flies, mosquitoes, rats and even sparrows, whose crime was supposed to lie in eating the grain and so depriving the populace of food. The following autumn, when a devastated harvest finally proved to Mao that the birds spent much more time eating the pests that destroyed grain than the grain itself, they were taken from the list. Unfortunately, the culling had been very thorough, and one of the things a visitor cannot fail to notice in China today is how few birds are to be seen.

In the newly emergent China, official policy now recognizes that Chairman Mao, the Great Helmsman of the nation, made the occasional navigational error. The estimate is set at 30 per cent errors, 70 per cent successes – a truly remarkable achievement in view of the devastated country he inherited. A Westerner who had lived many years in China before leaving in 1949, wrote on his return in 1966 that he looked in vain for the horribly deformed beggars, the distended stomachs of infants on the verge of starvation, the emaciated children defecating in the gutter, straining to expel nothing but tapeworms. All were gone. A new China had been created.

CHAPTER THREE
The Body as a Cosmos

The first principle of Chinese medicine, and every other aspect of Chinese thought, is yin and yang, the two opposing yet complementary sides of nature. Literally, the words mean the two banks of a river, one in the shade, the other in the sun. They represent the masculine and feminine, night and day, heat and cold.

Yang is masculine: sun, fire, heat, light, day, heaven and dryness. Yin is feminine: moon, night, earth, dampness and cold. Yang ascends. Yin descends. Yang is external, yin is internal. When they are in balance, the body is healthy. When imbalance occurs, illness results.

As civilization advanced in China, men began to study nature. Everything seemed to be in a perpetual state of transition. Winter gave way to spring, summer declined into autumn, flood followed drought, the skies clouded and cleared, day became night, planting led on to harvest, and so on throughout the universe. Nothing was constant, even the moon waxed and waned, and the planets came and went in the heavens.

Men also began to notice the effect of the seasons and the climate on general health. In winter, people were prone to colds and joint pains; in summer, the heat seemed to cause fevers. Closer study convinced them that not only did the weather have its effect on physical well-being, the human body seemed to have its own inner climate, precisely echoing nature. It, too, was in a constant circle of growth, development and decline.

To the Chinese, the human body is the cosmos in miniature. The universe is an organism and man is a microcosm of the universe. Just as the earth contains air, sea and land, the body has qi, fluids and blood. And just as the earth is governed by the seasons, so the body is affected by internal weather.

When constant rain saturates the earth it creates a swamp, where the ground is stagnant, swollen and spongy; when the body develops oedema, it is as a result of water retention, and the effect on the limbs is similar to what happens to the ground. And just as without rain, plants wilt and wither, so chapped hands and toes or cracked lips are brought about by inner dryness. Cold affects the circulation in the same way as ice freezes the waters of a stream. Heat is present in fever, red eyes, boils, sore throat or inflamed tissues.

Wind, too, can invade the body. The tremor which is characteristic of Parkinson's Disease, or the trembling symptoms following a stroke, are the result of wind evil, an internal climate affecting the organs: just as the leaves of a tree shiver and the branches sway in a high wind, so will the hands and the limbs when affected by this type of inner weather. Excess of heat may produce similar symptoms, in the way a blazing bonfire will create its own swirling wind.

Health is affected by both internal and external climates. External weather causes pathological changes in the human body. This is far from a uniquely oriental view: why else is bronchitis called 'the English disease'? How is it that winds like the mistral and the sirocco bring headaches? The Chinese have known for centuries that the pulse is affected by the seasons. Modern research has proved this to be the case.

Unlike the blood or body fluids, qi is an abstract concept. It cannot be seen, which is why Western medical science tends to reject its existence. Ancient texts refer to it as everything from a 'vital force' or 'subtle breath'. It is usually translated as a form of energy, a kind of well-spring of being which circulates through invisible channels in the body called meridians. In fact, everything in the cosmos has qi. Man himself is a form of qi. Breath is qi. Qi is the energy, the force, of creation. It is the body's defence mechanisms, and the oxygenator of the blood.

Similarly, in Chinese medicine, blood is not simply the red substance which circulates in the body and pours from a wound. It, too, has a non-material aspect and is generated and moved by qi. The fluids, which include sweat, saliva, gastric juices, urine and hormonal secretions, moisten the body and nourish the hair, skin, muscles and bone.

The concept of harmony is central to Chinese medicine; without it there can be no well-being. There are three harmonies:

1. **Harmony with nature.** The body must be in tune with the seasons. In springtime, when the days are lengthening, it is wise to take more exercise. In winter, with its cold weather and shorter days, people should follow the example of the animals and sleep more. The diet should also concentrate mainly on those foods which can be grown or harvested in each season.

2. **Internal harmony.** The five main organs, the heart, lungs, liver, spleen and kidneys should work in unison, as must the viscera with which they are paired. The main organs, called zhang, have a storage function. They are teamed with the viscera, the stomach, the gallbladder, the large and small intestines, and the bladder. These are the fu organs. They are hollow and have a transporting and transforming function. A sixth fu organ, also abstract, is called the 'triple burner' of the 'gate of life'. It is believed to be closely related to the kidney, and possibly refers to the adrenal gland. Each organ comes to the peak of its activity for only two hours at the same time each day.

3. **Mental and physical harmony.** If the physical condition is out of balance, the mental condition is wrong also. Emotional disturbance creates disharmony in the body: violent anger injures yang, and violent joy can do the same.

The ancient sages also compared the elements contained in nature with the main organs of the body, and paired them to demonstrate their interdependence and mutual reinforcement and restraint: fire for the heart, metal for the lungs, earth for the spleen, water for the kidneys and wood for the liver. These, in turn, are linked to different phases in a complex cosmic cycle. Fire is summer, the height of energy; wood represents growth and springtime; earth is the transitional period between the seasons, a kind of Indian summer; metal symbolizes autumn, the period of decline; and water denotes a resting state, similar to winter, or functions on the brink of change.

The use of the phrase 'five elements' to describe this theory is, strictly speaking, not correct. It is the result of a mistranslation, identifying a Chinese concept of transitional phases with the ancient Greek idea of the elements, but the use of the term has persisted for so long that it has become accepted and used even by the Chinese themselves. The true meaning, however, is the five transitional phases.

The interaction of the five elements

These concepts were first set out in the Chinese medical classic, the *Nei Jing* (see page 195), where their interaction was explained as follows:

Metal subjugates wood (an axe can cut down a tree).
Water subjugates fire (it will extinguish it).
Wood subjugates earth (tree roots penetrate the ground).
Fire subjugates metal (heat changes it from solid to liquid).
Earth subjugates water (it absorbs it).

Conversely:

Metal creates water (it turns to liquid when heated).
Water creates wood (rivers and rain feed trees).
Wood creates fire (as fuel).
Fire creates earth (it turns into ashes).
Earth creates metal (it is found underground).

This explains how one element aids or subdues another, and also explains the interdependence of the organs of the body. Since wood (which is linked to the liver) is nourished by water (which is linked to the kidney), the kidneys are the mother of the liver. Likewise, fire (which symbolizes the heart) is fed by wood, so the liver can nourish the heart.

If a patient develops heart trouble, a doctor will decide by his physical appearance which category his particular symptoms reveal. If he has a high colour, with purple lips, this is one indication that it is a condition of excess; the heart's fire is burning out of control, and treatment would involve the kidneys, since it is water which can dampen a fire. If, however, the patient's face is pale, this indicates deficiency. The fire is dangerously low and in need of fuel to restore it to brightness, thus – just as more wood is piled on a low fire – the liver would also be treated.

The organs are also interlinked with tastes, colours and climates, even with sounds, and all of these have some relevance to health and well-being. The tastes can influence the drugs which are prescribed, since every drug is defined according to one of five flavours. The sounds made by someone ill, not just the wheezing breath which comes with a respiratory complaint, but groaning or shouting, or even singing or unnatural laughter, will suggest the organ which is dysfunctioning. Some of these items are signs which will guide a doctor in his diagnosis. They are not inflexible, but, taken in total with the other symptoms, they can be useful indicators of a patient's condition.

Facial features are also paired. The heart is said to be 'open' to the tongue and paired with the small intestine; the lungs are open to the nose and paired with the large intestine; the liver is open to the eyes and paired with the gallbladder; the kidneys are open to the ears and paired with the bladder, and the spleen is open to the mouth and paired with the stomach.

- The organs also have a restraining and reinforcing effect on one another:
- The heart is connected with the pulse and ruled by the kidneys.
- The lungs are connected with the skin and ruled by the heart.
- The liver is connected with the tendons and ruled by the lungs.
- The spleen is connected with the flesh and ruled by the liver.
- The kidneys are connected with the bones and ruled by the spleen.

Also:

- The liver nourishes the muscles; the muscles strengthen the heart.
- The heart nourishes the blood; the blood strengthens the spleen.
- The spleen nourishes the flesh; the flesh strengthens the lungs.
- The lungs nourish the skin and hair; the skin and hair strengthen the kidneys.
- The kidneys nourish the bones and marrow; the bones and marrow strengthen the liver.

Table of relationships

Heart	Lungs	Liver	Kidney	Spleen
Tongue	Nose	Eyes	Ears	Mouth
Small Intestine	Large Intestine	Gallbladder	Bladder	Stomach
Fire	Metal	Wood	Water	Earth
Red	White	Green	Black	Yellow
Hot	Dry	Windy	Cold	Damp
Bitter	Pungent	Sour	Salt	Sweet
Laugh	Weeping	Shout	Groan	Sing

The five climates have a direct bearing on the organs:

- Heat injures the heart.
- Cold injures the lungs.
- Wind injures the liver.
- Damp injures the spleen.
- Dryness injures the kidneys.

The five flavours can cause physical harm, as follows:

- Excess of salt flavour hardens the pulse.
- Excess of bitter flavour withers the skin.
- Excess of pungent flavour knots the muscles.
- Excess of sour flavour toughens the flesh.
- Excess of sweet flavour causes aches in the bones.

In medical treatment, however:

- The salt flavour has a softening effect.
- The bitter flavour has a strengthening effect.
- The pungent flavour has a dispersing effect.
- The sour flavour has a gathering effect.
- The sweet flavour has a retarding effect.

The planets, numbers, animals, the five grains, the five fruits and the five points of the compass are all included in this numbers game, some of which are merely fanciful and added to conform to the sets of five. Each season was believed to originate from one point of the compass, but as there are only four directions and four seasons, the Centre and the Indian summer were introduced.

The heart is teamed with the planet Mars, with the South, with the number 7, the horse, the apricot, and glutinous rice.

The lungs are linked with Venus, the West, the dog, number 9, the pear, rice.

The liver is Jupiter, the East, chicken, number 8, the plum, and wheat.

The kidney is Mercury, the North, pig, six, chestnut, and beans.

The spleen is Saturn, the Centre, the cow, number 5, dates, and millet.

Although the five grains and the five fruits are listed as necessary components of the well-balanced daily diet, and were recommended by the Red Emperor in his famous book *The Great Herbal* (see page 196), the more arcane associations are probably additions from the early alchemists, rather than deriving from the more rigidly medical connections of the other elements.

The heart

This is the major organ in the blood circulatory system and therefore crucial to health. The Chinese call the heart the emperor of the body and say it is connected with heaven. It stores the spirit (shen), an abstract concept having some aspects of the Western meaning, as well as denoting general well-being both physical and mental. A healthy and robust person would be described as having shen in much the same way as we would describe somebody in a happy mood as being in good spirits. An unhealthy and lethargic person is considered to have 'bad shen'; not dissimilar to our description of someone in a gloomy mood as being in low spirits, although in Chinese terms the phrase refers to the physical as well as the mental state.

Like any emperor, the heart is protected by a guard, the pericardium, whose function it is to stop anything harmful getting through and attacking it. When the qi of the heart is weak, there will be circulation problems. Symptoms such as a purple face, or the purple toes and fingers caused by chilblains, are seen as a sign that the blood is stagnant and not circulating properly. The Chinese regard unconsciousness, coma or delirium as evidence that the spirit is disturbed, because heat, which is in the channels of the muscles, has invaded the blood and become trapped inside the pericardium.

The heart is open to the tongue, which is a good indicator of its condition. Indeed, the tongue plays a vital role in TCM diagnosis, since it is an internal organ that can be viewed from outside the body (the same is considered true of the eyes, since they are covered by lids) and is therefore an essential indicator of the internal condition. A red-tipped tongue can indicate insomnia, purple marks on it indicate poor circulation.

Western medicine has all the technology and very many effective drugs for heart problems, and a traditional Chinese doctor would suggest that a patient went first to a hospital for an ECG and check-up by Western cardiologists. Heart problems are often treated by a combination of both systems in China, because both offer very effective remedies.

Some mental illness is attributed to a heart–spirit problem. Schizophrenia is regarded as a problem of too much heat in the heart, so that the spirit is burnt, making sufferers restless and violent. The patient would be given medicines to calm the heart. Lotus seed sprouts are effective and cooling because the seeds come from the heart of the plant and the lotus grows in water.

Epilepsy is diagnosed as phlegm or dampness caused through a blocked heart meridian, which disturbs the spirit.

Conditions which are treated through the heart include coronary and artery disease, circulation problems, meningitis, mouth and tongue ulcers. Herbs which act on the heart include cinnamon twigs, red sage, aconite and lotus seed sprouts.

The lungs

Being next to the heart these are called the 'ministers'. They advise the emperor (the heart) and regulate his actions. The highest of the five organs in the body, they are very important as they dominate the qi. The lungs control breathing, inhaling and exhaling the air which is drawn from the heavens. They are believed to mix nutrition from the spleen (which is of the earth) with the air (which is from heaven) and spread it around the body, to aerate and moisturize. Lungs dominate the skin and the hair, and are open to the nose, the organ through which air is taken into the body.

The lungs have a descending function. The moisture which they are said to produce is comparable to mist, which sinks into the earth as water. This mist makes the joints more flexible and the muscles stronger, sending energy and water down to the kidneys to form urine. When the lungs function well, the hair grows in the same way as grass springs up after a shower of rain. Healthy, shining hair is one sign of strong lungs.

If the lung qi gets unbalanced, and travels upwards, the result will be coughing, sneezing and wheezing, plus stagnation of water, which is prevented from flowing downwards. This is the cause of puffy eyes in conditions such as influenza and tonsilitis.

When the lung energies are strong, the pores open and close easily. During very cold weather in China, people take ginger or spring onion 'tea' to help the lungs to open the pores and to expel cold from the body.

The lungs are open to the nose. A blocked or runny nose requires treatment through the lungs. Sneezing or hay fever are two conditions which are treated in the same way. A TCM doctor will prescribe herbs that help the lung energy to descend so that water moves, the pores open, and excess water can be flushed from the body without the use of too many diuretic drugs.

Conditions treated through the lungs include colds, influenza, asthma, bronchitis, nephritis, hay fever and oedema. The herbs often used include hot fennel root, lilyturf root, mulberry leaf and skullcap root.

The liver

The liver is the general of the army, in charge of stratagem and maintaining harmony or movement and evenness throughout the system. The smooth flow of qi is dependent upon the action of the liver, which stores the blood and adjusts its supply to meet the body's needs. Many blood problems are treated through the liver. If the qi and the blood are out of balance, the action of the liver will tune them.

Although the heart stores the spirit, it is the liver that can affect it. Any sudden change in the emotions may impair the flowing and dispersing function of the liver, while a disharmony in that organ will affect the emotional state, causing depression and a variety of mental problems ranging from anxiety to suicidal tendencies. This is diagnosed as liver stagnation.

Where Western physicians would prescribe anti-depressants, Chinese traditional doctors say that if the liver qi is made smooth and is moved, the depression will go. The Chinese pharmacopoeia includes herbs which can break the cycle of depression. There is also a well known medical formula used to treat emotional conditions, known as the Free and Easy Wanderer.

Stagnant liver energy results in heat and fermenting. Fire rises, causing anger, agitation, sleeplessness, headaches and dizziness. The Chinese term for this is gan ho, which is the origin of the English gung-ho, the phrase also used to describe hasty and sometimes ill-considered actions.

The liver also harmonizes the digestive system, helping the spleen and stomach to process food and drink, but if this fails, it can move in the wrong direction and enter the stomach and spleen in much the same way as an invading army, causing abdominal pain, nausea, belching, intestinal rumbling and diarrhoea.

The liver dominates the tendons, and the nails which are considered to be the ends of the tendons. When nails are fragile and brittle, it is attributed to liver weakness. Tendons, in TCM, include ligaments and sometimes muscles, so any stiffness or numbness there is considered to stem from the liver. It is open to the eyes. Itching, dry and red eyes are due to heat in the liver channel. Bright eyes characterize a harmonious spirit.

Conditions treated through the liver include gynaecological problems such as PMT, weight gain, stomach ache, gastric ulcers, cramp, stiffness of the joints, eye problems, depression and herpes. The herbs used include white peony root, Chinese angelica, thorowax root and Chinese gentian.

The kidneys

These dominate water, ridding the body of excess through the bladder and retaining 'good water' in the body, which is also thought to be the source of hormonal balance. The kidneys are said to store the essence of the being, and this is crucial to Chinese philosophy. It is concerned with inheritance, and is seen as something received genetically through one's parents. It is perhaps best explained as the Chinese concept of DNA.

Because it is a sacred gift from the ancestors, this essence must be treated with the utmost respect. It is referred to as 'before heaven' energy, that is to say, a gift bestowed on a child before birth, and it is finite. As life continues, it is gradually depleted by the ageing process, and if it is not treated with due deference at all times, the consequences can be serious. The body should never be abused by over-indulgence or any form of excess, from overwork to too much sex or drink. To do so, it is thought, will adversely affect every aspect not only of your own future, but possibly even the next generation's, since the weakness may be passed down to children.

A second pool of energy is also stored in the kidneys, and this is concerned with the constitution. In addition to producing urine, the kidneys absorb 'good' water and help it to vaporize. They are said to 'grasp' the air to help the lungs. The lungs may take in the air, but it is the kidneys that retain it in the body, to balance the function of breathing.

Thus when people grow old and their breathing becomes more shallow, this is attributed to kidney weakness. Some forms of asthma are treated by tonifying the kidneys, because although the condition is situated in the lung, it is said to be rooted in the kidney. Chinese medicine has had very encouraging results with some forms of asthma through tonifying the kidneys, though it must be stressed that this is a complex disease with various causes, not all of which respond to treatment.

Kidneys formulate the bone and marrow and nourish the hair and the teeth. Sharp hearing and strong teeth indicate strong kidneys.

The kidneys are open to the ears, the anus and the urethra. The ear is similar in shape to the kidney, as well as having an acupoint which covers every part of the body. Infertility treatment involves nourishing the kidneys and it is said that babies conceived through this treatment will be particularly strong because the mother's kidney energy has been strengthened.

Conditions treated include oedema, asthma (some forms), growth problems in children, deafness, tinnitus, bed-wetting, memory and concentration problems, infertility, backache. The herbs used include mulberry, mistletoe, eucommia bark, morinda root, cibot rhizome, dodder seeds.

The spleen

The Chinese concept of the human body is vastly different to the strictly anatomical view familiar to Westerners. Nowhere is this more apparent than in the matter of the spleen. In TCM, the spleen is in the centre of the body and fundamental to it in the same way as an axle is to a wheel. It is allied to the earth, and includes part of the liver, the pancreas and the stomach, and the small intestine.

The spleen transforms the vital force, qi, blood, food and drink to nourish the body. If it is not functioning properly, the body will be malnourished. A weak spleen is indicated by poor appetite, poor digestion, fatigue, anaemia, tiredness and weakness.

Water prevented from leaving the body can cause damp, resulting in diarrhoea, weight gain and feelings of heaviness.

Blood is pushed by the heart and stored by the liver, but spleen energy keeps it flowing. An illness with symptoms involving any bleeding would be attributed to spleen deficiency. It is connected to the stomach and works in unison with it.

Spleen energy moves up, nourishing the brain; stomach energy moves down, keeping the bowels open. Should spleen energy descend, prolapse of organs such as the kidneys, uterus or anus can occur. Overeating or eating the wrong foods can result in the stomach energy rising, causing vomiting, bowel changes or acid regurgitation.

Since the spleen generates energy and blood, it controls the muscles and limbs. The spleen is open to the mouth, influencing appetite and taste. Research in China has established a link between the spleen and the immune system. Tonifying the spleen raises the blood cell count, particularly white cells, and combats infection.

Conditions treated include general weakness and lassitude, diarrhoea, anaemia, obesity, multiple sclerosis. The herbs used include ginger, liquorice, tangerine peel, peony root, ginseng, Chinese angelica, astragalus.

CHAPTER FOUR
A Very Peculiar Practice?

One of the Chinese doctors who teaches TCM to students at a college in Reading, Berkshire, has a favourite device to demonstrate the accuracy of the four diagnostic methods which are at the foundation of traditional practice. He sends a student into an anteroom with a new patient to gather all the details of his or her medical history, before the patient goes into the consulting room to be examined.

Then, without access to the medical notes, and faced with a patient he is seeing for the first time, of whom he knows nothing, and of whom he has asked no questions, the doctor will make his examination, diagnose the complaint, and summarize the patient's medical history from his own clinical observations. The accuracy of his findings often astonishes his students.

Very few physical secrets are hidden from a vigilant TCM doctor. Through the ancient skill of pulse-reading, a trained and experienced practitioner can detect not merely the condition of the patient, but often the medication he or she has taken, and even their emotional state.

The students at the Berkshire college thought their teacher had been caught out when he remarked to one woman that she was taking a contraceptive pill. The patient denied this, but the doctor insisted. Had she not taken it in the past? Yes indeed, but that was five years ago, she said, and she hardly thought it worth mentioning after that length of time. According to the doctor, the effect of several years on the pill was still detectable in her body. He could pick up the signals merely by reading her pulse. Another patient was even more surprised when his TCM doctor asked him if there had been some trouble earlier that day. Taken aback, he admitted there had been a row with a work colleague that morning. How did she know? Ah, because his liver pulse was showing anger, she told him.

Good guesswork or magical diagnostic techniques? Most Westerners would unhesitatingly opt for the first explanation, but experienced TCM doctors will insist that neither is correct; to them it is simply sound clinical practice. They do not merely count how fast the heart is beating, or whether the patient has high or low blood pressure, by pulse-reading. Each organ has a pulse of its own, and each pulse has a variety of patterns that can be read like a book. The liver function is always affected by anger, and this is immediately identified in the pulse of that organ, just as the effects of the birth pill are apparent in the general pulse pattern of the entire body. The doctor described the pulse beat in such cases as wavy and soft, indicating a hormone imbalance. Strictly speaking, no wavy category is listed in the medical classics. The practitioner's long experience had taught him to recognize the signals indicating the presence of chemical drugs in the system. Artificial substances all make their own impression on the pulse tone. Only long years in practice will teach the physician how to recognize the indications of each.

When we remember the restrictions under which doctors had to work in olden times, the refinement which the Chinese have brought to the science of pulse diagnosis is more easily appreciated. A court physician could not examine the women of the emperor's household. No man except the eunuchs who guarded their quarters was allowed to look upon them. A doctor could venture no closer than the curtains which veiled the sick woman's bed. She would then extend an arm through the draperies, and diagnosis and treatment would rest entirely on what the practitioner was able to discern through her pulse. If his diagnosis and subsequent treatment were not correct, woe betide him.

Similar skill was demonstrated in defining the patient's emotional state through his pulse. Even in present-day China, it is not done to show emotion. Strangers who give way to expressions of anger will merely amuse any onlookers. Nobody is being rude. It is simply considered that outbursts of temper result in a damaged liver and a loss of dignity. Who would be so foolish as to risk either? The Chinese habitually hide their emotions, but that is not to say they are unaffected by them. Friends and neighbours may not be aware of a person's inner feelings, but they cannot be hidden from his TCM doctor.

As soon as a patient walks into his surgery, a TCM doctor starts assessing his or her physical and mental condition. The way she walks and carries herself, the slope of the shoulders, the expression on her face. Even the sound of the voice and the manner of speaking will tell the alert and sensitive physician something about the state of the patient. These are valuable indicators of general health, and a full picture of the patient's well-being can be built up without using a stethoscope, testing the blood pressure, or taking a blood or urine sample. All that a TCM doctor needs to use to get the same kind of information, are the four diagnostic methods: looking, listening and smelling (the words for both are the same in Chinese), asking and palpating.

The early doctors had no means of measuring or analysing the chemical composition of body fluids, and it was through observation and clinical experience that they gradually evolved a system which gave them reliable information about the patient's health. The accuracy was such that the same methods continue to be used today.

TCM doctors working in the West, and in hospitals like the one at Tianjin which use a combination of the two therapies, can always confirm their findings by laboratory tests, when they consider it necessary, and frequently do so. But as a general rule, the more experienced a TCM practitioner is, the more he can tell about a patient's condition at the initial examination.

Some of the famous medical sages of old taught that the very best doctor should be able to identify the illness simply by studying the patient's physical appearance, the second best would also use listening and smelling, and so on. That is not to say that any doctor would take one long look at a patient and pronounce on his disorder without further ado, although gifted physicians like Bian Que were apparently able to do so. It simply means that the expert diagnostician should be able to discern the illness at first glance. If he is good at his work, he should then be able to confirm that first opinion by completing all four examinations.

The modern Chinese doctor will use the four diagnostic methods, and in addition he or she sometimes has all the usual equipment of a Western doctor's surgery, stethoscope included, though they use it mainly to reassure Western patients, who can follow their own progress much more easily if, for example, their blood pressure is monitored in the orthodox way. The traditional method of taking a pulse can diagnose high blood pressure just as effectively, however; and more besides.

Western doctors are also taught the importance of observation and the signs they can read in the physical appearance of the patient. They note the complexion, check the state of the tongue, the brightness of the eyes and the condition of the skin, but these tend to be secondary aspects to the information they glean through taking blood pressure, and listening to the heartbeat and respiration.

Yet before the appropriate equipment became available, doctors in the West also relied more on the evidence of their own eyes. At the turn of the century, a celebrated physician who taught at Edinburgh University was noted for the acuteness of his observation. Like the TCM doctor in Reading, he loved to give new students a demonstration of how much could be learned by close attention to detail. An unknown patient would enter his surgery, the consultant would make his physical examination silently, ask the patient to return to the waiting room, and then invite the students to tell him all the information they had gleaned from that brief examination.

One day a particularly impressionable undergraduate was assisting at his hospital clinic when a new patient walked painfully into the surgery on swollen legs. When the man had left the room again, the consultant asked the student what he had learned about the patient from the physical examination.

After letting him fumble for words for a while, the consultant gave his own assessment: the man had elephantiasis, a tropical disease which meant that he had lived abroad at some point. His clothes and accent revealed him to be working-class. He was polite and pleasant, with a quiet air of self-confidence, but he did not remove his hat when he entered the room, as a normally courteous person of his type would do automatically in a doctor's surgery. This suggested he was an army man, since soldiers do not remove their caps indoors. His relaxed and confident bearing suggested that he was used to some authority. Here, surely, was a sergeant, who had made the army his career and had probably spent much of it in the tropics. Elementary, my dear Watson!

It was a lesson in the importance of observation which the student never forgot. In later life, when he turned to writing, the incident led to the creation of the most famous detective in fiction. The prototype for Sherlock Holmes was his old professor. It is doubtful whether there are many Western doctors who use such highly developed powers of observation in this age of high technology, but a Chinese doctor follows his ancient craft based on the same procedures as his forefathers. No matter what technology can offer in the way of diagnostic aids, his first and most valued diagnostic tools lie in his own training.

In TCM, the tongue is one of the most vital indicators of health problems, and learning to read its signs is a science in itself. Because the tongue is inside the body but can be viewed externally, its value as a diagnostic tool is immense. In the College of Traditional Medicine in Beijing, there is a special room in which are stored wax specimens of tongues of all varieties, showing signs of internal disorders. The tongue size, shape, moisture, colour, movement and the quality of its coating are all indications to a Chinese doctor of the state of the internal organs.

The tip of the tongue is the location for the heart and lung; if it has fissures, furrows or wrinkles the doctor will interpret this as a sign that there is something wrong in one or other of those organs. The edge of the tongue shows the condition of the liver and gallbladder, the spleen and stomach are set in the centre, and the kidney is located at the root. Any enlargement of the taste buds at the root of the tongue will indicate heat in the genital system or the urinary bladder. A female patient with this symptom, plus a pronounced red colour in the tongue, will possibly suffer from menstrual problems or bladder trouble.

A swollen tongue indicates excessive fire of the heart or accumulated heat in the heart or the spleen. A plump tongue with teeth-prints on the lower border suggests a deficiency of the spleen and kidney. If the spleen is not functioning properly, it leads to retention of water, causing the tongue to swell and become compressed by the teeth. A patient who constantly licks his or her lips may be suffering from internal dryness of the spleen and stomach.

Listening involves noting the quality of the voice and the patient's speech pattern, whether the voice is hoarse or a whisper, weak or hesitant, or firm and clear. The odours the doctor looks for will vary according to the nature of the complaint; the quality of the odours themselves can be difficult to describe, and is based on ancient teaching and experience.

A TCM doctor practising in Europe has to adjust his sensory perceptions to Western culture. The Chinese do not smother themselves in scents, highly perfumed lotions and deodorants as we tend to do. Nor do they eat dairy products, which they say give those who have recently eaten them a strong characteristic smell. Any subtle body odour in Western patients may well be masked by a plethora of toiletries, and overlaid by last night's quiche. Nevertheless there are still olfactory signs which can be valuable pointers to the doctor in confirming his diagnosis.

Excessive heat will be characterized by a fetid smell and has associations with digestive disorders. Pungent and fishy odour indicates pathogenic infection inside the organs, caused by cold-dampness and deficiency syndrome. If the patient's vomit contains pus and blood and has a fishy smell, he is possibly suffering from a pulmonary abscess. The scent of rotten apples suggests serious diabetes mellitus.

The interrogative examination involves the patient's description of his symptoms and medical history. Details of his age, occupation, place of birth, his living conditions and environment, his hobbies and habits, even his dreams and his childhood ailments, would all be taken into consideration. The age of the parents if living, or their age and the cause of death, are obviously relevant in the case of inherited disease. Therefore medical details of siblings and family diseases will also be sought.

Palpating reveals the condition of the skin; whether it is moist, dry, hot or cold. Pain may be increased or alleviated by pressure, and this will help the doctor to decide whether the ailment is an excess or a deficiency condition. In TCM, all illness stems from imbalance. Pain which is alleviated by warmth, and eased by pressure, indicates deficiency in problems connected with the stomach and the digestive system. When touch makes the pain worse, as in appendicitis or gastroenteritis, it is likely to be caused by an excess.

The pulse is perhaps the most important of these examinations, so much so that when a Chinese patient feels in need of medical attention he or she doesn't say, 'I'm going to see the doctor,' but, 'I'm going to have my pulses read.' While he does this, the doctor will ask the patient to rest both wrists in turn on a small cushion, and will then take the pulse by resting three fingers on the radial artery at specified points, called the cun, guan and chi, or the inch, bar and cubit.

On the left wrist, the index finger detects patterns from the heart and small intestine; the second finger from the liver and gallbladder; the third from the kidney and bladder. At each location the doctor will read three times, lightly at first with what is called a 'touching' manner; then with moderate pressure, called 'searching'; finally he will probe firmly between the muscle and the bone, and this is called 'pressing'. The different force of each touch will enable him to detect changes in the pulse condition. One patient described the procedure very graphically by saying she 'felt as if the doctor was practising the piano on my wrist'.

The right wrist reveals the pattern of the lung and large intestine, the spleen and the stomach, and what is called the 'gate of life' or sometimes the 'fire of the vital gate' (this is a metaphysical secondary organ which is believed to be closely related to the kidney, physiologically and pathologically, and is a function connected with the production of adrenalin).

Each rhythm is then defined. A pulse can be wiry, choppy, empty, deep, or any one of twenty-eight categories, some of which require immense skill to detect. Medical students will be taught how to recognize a floating pulse because it can be felt with a light touch, but grows fainter on pressing hard: in olden times, it was compared to wood floating on water. A slippery pulse is likened to feeling beads on a plate.

These readings will tell the practitioner about the state of both the body and the mind, because the two have always been inseparable in TCM theory. The link between stress and illness may be a relatively recent concept to us in the West, but not in TCM which holds not only that disease can result from emotional factors, but that each emotion is connected to a particular organ, and will influence its function. Paradoxically, the Chinese do not go in for psychology as a separate discipline. They do not pay much attention to concepts such as the subconscious, the ego or the id. The organs will reveal all they need to know, without probing the psyche.

This is particularly useful since the Chinese are a private and reticent people, and do not consider it polite to discuss their personal emotional problems even with the family doctor. In any event, the doctor would not ask such questions. There is a Chinese proverb much the same as the English adage about not washing your dirty linen in public. But there is no need for the practitioner to delve into the private lives of his patients. While he sits quietly listening to a pulse for five or ten minutes much is communicated to him about his patient's state of mind.

There are of course conditions in the modern world where a patient needs to be encouraged to talk about his or her feelings to reveal the real causes of anorexia or obsessional behaviour, for example, and then the TCM doctor may suggest that the patient seek psychiatric treatment elsewhere. But there are many examples of depressive illness which can be treated with acupuncture and herbal medicine. Some herbs are extremely effective at breaking the cycle of depression.

Merely holding the wrist will indicate whether the person is tense or nervous, or relaxed. The pulse will indicate the precise emotional state because a different organ is affected in each case. The doctor can feel fear and shock in the kidney pulse, because in TCM the kidney also includes the adrenal glands sited above it. In Western medicine, we acknowledge that adrenalin is triggered in the primitive 'fight or flight' mechanism which is a reflex action in all frightening situations. In Chinese medicine, the heart may also be affected, because the spirit resides there, and could be disturbed by the experience.

Even feelings of joy – the emotion linked to the heart – can damage that organ if excessive. This is not so far-fetched as it sounds. A pools winner could become so overcome by his unexpected good fortune that the excitement might bring on a heart attack. Someone who has suffered a serious loss, or is brooding over a problem, may be so preoccupied that he or she does not eat properly, thereby injuring the spleen, which has the function of transforming food into energy. That effect can be read by a TCM doctor in the spleen pulse.

If somebody is in an anxiety state, breathing may quicken, he or she may begin to chain-smoke, or become reclusive and refuse to leave the house, not getting sufficient fresh air and thereby affecting the function of the lungs. This will come through in his lung pulse. Someone who is terrified may lose bladder control, another example of how shock or fear can affect kidney function.

Pulse-reading has evolved through the centuries, as anatomical knowledge advanced. The *Nei Jing* mentioned many types of pulse but there is confusion over the meaning of some names, and one school of thought in modern China suspects that in the case of the more arcane categories, the ancient physicians may have enjoyed the aura of superior knowledge this gave them, although there are many highly qualified TCM doctors working in Britain who insist that they can detect not only pregnancy in a woman's pulse, but even the sex of the child. They believe that the rarer pulse tones mentioned in ancient manuscripts are probably not understood because they have not been translated properly.

Whatever the truth of the matter, the information a present-day TCM doctor can glean from this training in pulse-reading will still seem baffling to most Westerners. There is nothing about it which cannot be readily explained, however, and to think of it as in any way mysterious is to do TCM a disservice.

For example, medical scientists at Shandong Medical College were able to confirm the TCM theory that the pulse alters with the variation of the seasons by measuring the pulse of over 1,000 healthy volunteers, using sophisticated equipment for measuring heart pulse called a sphygmoelectrocardiograph machine. Further sphygmogram research revealed that a slippery pulse developed twenty minutes after drinking wine or water, because the blood volume increases. A taut pulse was traced after the subjects put their feet into icy water. The cold contracted the blood vessels of the skin, increasing the blood pressure and muscular tension.

Traditional medicine may be an ancient science, but it has survived because it keeps pace with medical progress. Despite the fact that there were no such things as cortisone or steroids when the *Nei Jing* was compiled, or when the other celebrated medical textbook, the *Mai Jing*, or Pulse Classic, was written about AD 280, a skilled TCM doctor can readily detect drugs such as these, because the medical theory he is taught has kept pace with modern practice, and present-day researchers have further refined pulse-reading to take account of twentieth-century medical advances, by clinical study and day-to-day practice and observation.

Because traditional medicine is a system foreign to Western eyes, there is a considerable degree of misunderstanding of how it works, which even extends to highly qualified Western doctors who do not hesitate to use acupuncture in their own clinics.

Chinese doctors know exactly how it works, but then they have the concept of qi, the invisible force which governs not just the human body but the whole planetary system. The West may believe that qi cannot be seen, analysed, measured or detected, but in TCM the qi within the human body is the oxygenator of the blood and as such its presence in the system can be readily detected by means of modern medical equipment.

A brief summary of Chinese traditional practice, with its talk of qi and syndromes of heat and stagnation does perhaps sound simplistic and unscientific on first hearing, and unfortunately a first hearing is very often all it will get from modern science and medicine. Ironically, too, the natural accessibility of TCM may have been a stumbling block to its acceptance in the West as a science. As previously mentioned, medical men in China did not evolve a language of their own to describe their findings. They saw no point in blinding patients with science, so they explained their diagnosis, treatment and the nature of disease in everyday terminology which every patient could understand.

They still do in mainland China, although the descriptions they use may sound a little strange to Western ears.

Qualified TCM doctors coming over from China now have a solid grounding in allopathic medicine as well as their own system, so they continue the practice of using language with which the patient is familiar. A Western patient is perfectly well aware that if her feet and ankles swell through water retention, the medical term for the condition is oedema. If that is what is wrong, the TCM doctor will say so, in order for there to be no misunderstanding between them.

In his own terms, he may start treating the spleen so that the 'evil dampness' will disappear, because the spleen's function is to regulate and irrigate the body fluids. When it is not working properly, the patient will suffer aching, abdominal distension, feelings of heaviness and urination deficiencies. In China, a patient would understand perfectly when told his body must be helped to expel the 'evil dampness'. To Western ears, the process might sound like something straight out of a scene in *The Exorcist*.

Once a patient's problems have been diagnosed, a TCM doctor will prescribe acupuncture, herbs, or if necessary manipulation, osteopathy, and sometimes qi gong exercises. It would be far too confusing, in any event, to offer a traditional description of the ailment, since where Western medicine recognizes only one disease in six patients, a TCM doctor may identify six different patterns of disharmony, with a different diagnosis in each case.

In a Western hospital, six patients suffering with shingles would be diagnosed as suffering from the same complaint, and receive the same treatment. In a TCM ward, six different patterns of disharmony might be detected. Someone suffering an outbreak of shingles on the upper body has a different dysfunction from someone whose spots are confined to the legs and feet. Every patient is treated individually and holistically. The herbal remedies given to each would be adjusted accordingly, although (in the case of a heart patient, for example) they will all contain herbs which are effective in treating the disease that a cardiologist would call coronary artery disease. The TCM doctor will use exactly the same term when discussing the case with the patient.

A good example of how treatment methods vary between Western and TCM practice is provided by the real-life case of a fifty-seven-year-old school teacher who contracted encephalitis. The illness started with migraine-type headaches, and her GP eventually sent her to hospital, where myalgic encephalomyelitis (ME) was diagnosed. She was put on intravenous antibiotics three times a day for ten days, but after three weeks with no sign of an improvement she discharged herself.

Unable to recognize written words, unable to concentrate, and without co-ordination, this patient was very depressed about the future in addition to feeling extremely ill. Because she had undergone successful TCM treatment for arthritis in the past, she decided to seek help from the same doctor to see if Chinese medicine offered any better hope of a cure.

His examination showed that her pulse was floating and soft, without pulse energy. The floating nature meant that the exterior of her body was affected by the disease, the soft pulse indicated insufficiency of blood and poor vital energy. Her facial colour showed a lack of lustre, with pale lips, meaning that the patient was very weak and emotional. Her tongue substance was reddened, with a thick furry yellow coating, indicating inward heat penetration.

The TCM treatment consisted of three weekly sessions over the next six months, acupuncture being used to treat the symptoms and relieve the headaches, and herbal medicine to cure the virus. It included moutain p'i (tree peony bark) which cools the blood, improves the circulation and treats the fever. After six weeks, the patient's vision was normal and she was able to drive again. The headaches, irritability and insomnia were still present, but by this time her pulse, which the doctor read as 'forceful' showed that her defensive energy had not been damaged by the illness.

The tongue was a paler shade of red, with lighter yellow furring, indicating that the symptoms which were originally internal were now external. After two months, her visits to the doctor were cut to twice a week, and finally to once a week. The pulse had become moderate, the fur on the tongue was much lighter, and the substance a healthy, pinkish red.

By August, the patient was able to read once more, and at Christmas she was able to go back to full-time teaching. In Western terminology, her encephalitis was cured. In TCM terms, she had been given treatment to enable her own body to fight a syndrome of blood stasis and poor vital energy.

There is another marked difference in attitude between the two systems. In olden days, Chinese patients paid their doctor to supervise their well-being on a permanent basis, and to see to it that they stayed healthy. To some extent, they still follow this custom. Most Westerners will hesitate to consult a doctor when they merely feel 'off colour', because they don't want to waste his or her time. This is the very point at which a TCM doctor prefers his patient to consult him. He sees his job as preventing illness from taking a hold by picking up the early signs, and so do his patients. Therefore they consult him before trouble starts in earnest.

Westerners familiar with TCM often come to follow the same routine, visiting their Chinese doctor merely when they feel a little out of sorts. He will examine them to locate the source of the trouble and give treatment to prevent the illness from developing. He is often also likely to suggest continuing treatment after what Westerners would consider a cure. This is because a TCM doctor does not consider the work done until he has reached the root of the ailment. An abscess is not cured merely because it has burst and the skin has healed. If it has been caused by internal heat and fire poison, then treatment will continue until the source of the heat is expelled from the organs, otherwise the trouble could recur.

It helps to understand this approach if you are consulting a TCM practitioner for the first time. A good doctor will explain in Western terms what the trouble is, and he may also explain, if the patient is interested, what the traditional diagnosis is, and how he will go about treating the condition. Don't be afraid to ask for an idea of how long the treatment may last. Obviously, no doctor can predict precisely when a condition will be cured, but a TCM doctor will be able to say whether the treatment will be long- or short-term, and he will certainly be able to tell you whether or not the condition is likely to respond to acupuncture and herbs.

All private medical treatment is expensive. By comparison with orthodox medical practice, or some of the alternative and complementary therapies on offer nowadays, TCM tends to be in the moderate to middle price range. Ask at the outset what the charges for a consultation will be, what is the expected duration of treatment, and the cost of the medicine.

In China, patients frequently see the doctor every day in the early course of their illness, so that he can monitor their progress closely and adapt his prescription to the changing condition of the patient. Obviously, the more intensive the treatment and the more closely the patient's progress is monitored, the quicker the cure. In Britain, TCM doctors usually like to see patients at least once a week until the condition starts to show definite signs of improvement, after which visits may be cut down to once a fortnight, then once a month, or once every two or three months, until the source of the illness has been reached.

A Chinese doctor ensures that his patient is in good physical shape before he is satisfied. If you consult a TCM doctor for the first time, bear this in mind. Many Western patients stop treatment as soon as the symptoms disappear, and TCM doctors understand this, but if you build up a good relationship with the doctor, and ask him to explain your progress and his prognosis at each visit, you will be able to make your own judgement about whether you feel it is worthwhile continuing treatment until the doctor is satisfied that he has cured the root cause and the condition will not return. From a medical viewpoint, it almost certainly will be, but understandably the financial aspect has to be taken into account.

Try to ensure that the physician you consult has good credentials. A piece of paper written in Chinese characters is no guarantee of a sound university training. If you can't read it, it isn't telling you anything. Most patients find their way to Chinese practitioners through personal recommendation, and this is by far the most satisfactory method, though there are organizations whose members are trained to set standards (see page 204).

Some members have been taught in colleges in the UK, and they may not have the intensive training and clinical experience that a properly qualified doctor receives in the medical colleges of his homeland, although all will have reached a reliable level of competence, and some will also be qualified in aspects of Western medicine, perhaps as nurses or physiotherapists. If you require reassurance, contact the college where the doctor studied.

In Britain at present, anyone can set up consulting rooms to practise any form of complementary medicine. Responsible practitioners who care for the reputation of their profession set up their own regulatory boards, and have them officially registered. This gives the client some protection, and enables the members who belong to the organization to be covered by insurance. There are organizations in this country for TCM practitioners, but not all practitioners are members. This does not necessarily indicate that they are not up to the required standard, although in some instances it may do so, which is why it is always wise to check with the register to ensure that the doctor concerned has not been turned down by the association. Some doctors, however, feel that their qualifications are higher than the standards set by organizations in the West, and for that reason choose not to belong. It is therefore particularly important to make as many inquiries as possible about the doctor you plan to see.

A good, established doctor will have a known reputation. He or she will be happy to work alongside a Western GP. They will not interfere with the medicine which the patient is already taking from their GP or hospital; certainly not until such time as the patient's condition has improved significantly. However, their treatment is always geared towards helping the body's own immune system to help itself, and they prefer to get patients to a point, as early as possible, where steroids, cortisone and other strong drugs can be discontinued, as they regard them (in common with most Western doctors) as injurious to the immune system in the long term.

They will always refer a patient to a Western doctor or hospital if they diagnose a problem which requires surgery, special tests or clinical investigation. Good Chinese doctors are anxious to share their skills with Western colleagues and co-operate on cases, but all too often they get scant encouragement, and occasionally their methods are dismissed as hocus pocus. This is not only insulting to them, but also frequently means lost opportunities for health care.

Chinese traditional medicine has many strengths which Western medicine lacks, but the reverse is equally true. As a general rule, TCM is strongest in treating chronic conditions, and Western medicine is best at coping with acute cases. When the two systems work in harmony, the ideal balance is achieved.

The pulse rhythms

Among the things a doctor can detect from pulse-reading are the four categories of disease: whether the condition is yin or yang, internal or external, caused by cold or heat, excess or deficiency. The doctor reads both wrists, using three fingers. Each organ has its own pulse which can be felt at a particular point. On the right hand:

First finger indicates the lung and large intestine.
Second finger picks up the pulse of the spleen and stomach.
Third finger reads the pulse of the left kidney and the 'life gate' (the adrenal function which is part of the kidney in TCM).

On the left hand:

First finger indicates the heart and pericardium and small intestine.
Second finger locates the pulse of the liver and gallbladder.
Third picks up the pulse of the right kidney and the urinary bladder.

Internal or external

Fo Floating pulse. Apparent without pressure. Indicates an internal and minor ailment.
Chen Sinking pulse. Has to be pressed very hard. Indicates an interior illness.
Medium Indicates a normal, healthy person.

Cold or heat

Su Rapid. More than four beats, indicating heat.

Thousands of years ago, Chinese doctors were taught that there should be four beats in a patient's pulse in the time it took him to breathe in and out. That technique is still used, now confirmed by Western medicine which says that an average pulse beats eighteen times to one minute. Multiply that by 4, and you have 72, the normal pulse rate.
Huang Slow. Less than four beats, indicating cold and weakness.

Deficiency or excess

Hsi Excessive. A strong pulse which will not disappear even under pressure. Indicates abnormal energy such as the lungs gasping for breath in pneumonia

Xu Deficiency. A weak pulse which will disappear under slight pressure. Indicates a weakness of qi and blood.

Pulse shape (can be measured by a pulse machine, like an ECG)

Xuan Wiry like a string of a violin. Tight. Indicates stagnation of qi, damp, phlegm and pain.

Hua Slippery like pebbles rolling on a plate. Indicates phlegm and damp, also indicates pregnancy.

Jin Extremely tight like middle of the rope in a tug of war. Indicates cold and wind.

Chang Long pulse. Can be detected beyond the length of three fingers. Indicates qi and blood are in good condition, or may suggest excessive heat. (A doctor will judge how fast it is and take other examinations into account.)

Duan Short pulse. Means weakness of qi or blockage of qi and blood.

Hong Full pulse, like a tide flooding in. Indicates excessive heat and damp.

Ko Empty. Feels hollow like pressing finger on the neck of a spring onion. Indicates heavy bleeding and blood deficiency.

Se Choppy. Like scraping bamboo with a small knife. Indicates a blood deficiency and yin deficiency.

Xi Thready. Very thin line. Indicates weakness of blood and yin deficiency. Can also be qi deficiency.

There are many other pulse rhythms – irregular pulse, heat in the pulse, moving pulse, and so on – including some which are not in the ancient books but have been identified in recent times as indicating chemical drugs in the system. Those listed above are the basics.

CHAPTER FIVE
From the Casebook

It is a platitude of the modern age to say that man has landed on the moon but still cannot cure the common cold. No matter how much knowledge the human race has accrued in these days of often miraculous scientific advance, we have a long way to go before medicine of any kind, including our own familiar allopathic variety, can successfully cure all ailments.

Colds we may have to put up with for a year or two yet, but flu is a different matter. Chinese medicine doesn't use words like bacteria or virus, but it has herbs to treat them, and doctors have a number of ingredients in their pharmacopoeia which modern research has shown to be capable of breaking the viral structure. Some of the influenza strains can be treated with prescriptions which have been in existence for centuries, and which Chinese people buy over the counter at home, and at Chinese herbal shops and supermarkets in Britain.

Ordinary Chinese people are steeped in a culture which regards a basic grasp of medical knowledge as fundamental to life, and they absorb information about their own qi, yin and yang, deficiency and excess, with their mother's milk. They usually treat simple ailments themselves.

If they have something more serious, or chronic, they will naturally seek out a doctor, either a Western-style practitioner or a TCM doctor, according to choice. Increasingly, as China's open-door policy brings an exchange of knowledge and understanding, we in the West have access to traditional herbal medicine too.

The two systems have precisely the same aim, but reach it by different methods. It often happens that what one method is not 100 per cent successful in treating can be cured more effectively by the other. For the purposes of this chapter, we will concentrate on conditions where TCM seems to offer a better hope of cure or relief than allopathic medicine.

Ankylosis spondylitis

The patient, Mrs P., had suffered from the disease for three years before seeking TCM treatment. Anti-inflammatory tablets helped to keep her mobile and reduce the pain and discomfort, and she followed the Hay diet, but her condition was deteriorating. Conventional medical advice included eating a lot of protein. The TCM doctor, however, suggested a diet free of dairy produce, with very little red meat, particularly beef.

Mrs P.'s pulse was defined as 'fine' (indicating exhaustion of the vital essence and body fluids) and 'rapid' (meaning internal heat) and her tongue substance was reddened with a dry top and a slimy coating. The condition of her tongue indicated poor constructive and inborn energy and showed retention of body fluids.

After the first treatment with acupuncture and herbal medicine, she stopped taking the anti-inflammatory pills, and this forty-four-year old patient continued to visit the surgery near her Reading home twice weekly for lengthy acupuncture sessions, as her physical condition continued to improve.

'Sometimes I had needles in my hands, or my neck – each area had to be treated separately and took time, but I got immense relief from the sessions, and also from the herbs.

'I had a history of cold sores on the lips, which Dr Lee always got very concerned about. He said it was most important to treat them. They took a while to clear up, but I don't have them now. He also predicted a hormonal imbalance, which he said could cause problems at the menopause, and some of the herbal medicine he gave me was intended to regulate my blood and so avoid difficulties later on.'

The patient made such good progress that she was able to stop attending the doctor, but unfortunately some months later, she caught a virus which affected her spondilitis badly. 'I got cystitis, and a second very severe bout of spondylitis, affecting my arms, neck, hands and one shoulder joint as well as my spine, so I had to go back to my GP for the anti-inflammatory drugs, although Dr Lee did not approve of me taking them, but I couldn't get to work without them, and if I couldn't work, I couldn't have my TCM treatment every week.

'The sessions are not at all expensive in terms of the wonderful care I receive. I pay £20 each session and that includes treatment which often lasts six hours, but the family budget is tight, and it is because I work that I can afford it.'

'It has taken five months of herbal medicines and acupuncture since my last attack, and I am now down from three pills a day to one every other day. The improvement is continuing and the TCM doctor is pleased with my progress, so I hope I shall not have to take the drugs for much longer.'

The patient is on a strict diet with no red meat. She steams the fish and chicken she is allowed, and eats a lot of green vegetables. Her tongue is a healthy pinkish red, with a coating of white fur with saliva, showing that the body fluids are in balance again. Her pulse has changed to moderate with pulse energy, as her general condition continues to improve.

'My GP encourages me to keep up the acupuncture, which he knows is helping me enormously. He raised his eyebrows when I told him about the herbs, but I told him I have absolute faith in Dr Lee. I know I am in capable hands, and feel that the medicine he prescribes is doing its work.'

Asthma

A persistent, extremely bad cough which lasted for weeks on end and didn't respond to any of the patent or prescribed medicines, finally persuaded Oliver's mother that there was something more serious underlying her little boy's condition. The family GP agreed, and referred the eight-year-old to an asthma specialist, who said the condition was certainly asthma-related. She prescribed antibiotics to clear up an infection and gave the boy an inhaler. Oliver's mother asked if it might not be appropriate to give allergy tests to confirm the diagnosis, but the doctor was adamant that these were not necessary.

The thought of starting her son on an inhaler so early in his life worried Oliver's mother. She felt he might become dependent on it, and that he would never be able to take part in sports or to run about with the other children in his school. The day after he started his course of antibiotics, she took him for acupuncture treatment.

'Driving over in the car I was a bit worried at the thought of having needles stuck in me,' Oliver admits. But when he met Lorna, she gave him such confidence that by the time he got on the couch, he wasn't worried any more.

The treatment made him feel numb in some of the acupoints, and gave him pins and needles in his feet. 'It wasn't comfortable, but it didn't worry me at all. When I finished the treatment, I felt really good. It was a great feeling.'

He completed the course of pills from the Western doctor, and had an acupuncture session once a week for five weeks. He has never used the inhaler, and his tonsils, which were very swollen and sore, were treated by Dr Hsu on a subsequent visit.

'She put the needle in my throat under my chin, and it was a really peculiar feeling. My throat started to hurt and I could hardly move my jaw. Then I felt something happening, as if my tonsil was shrinking.' It was. When his mother examined his throat later, the swelling had gone down.

'I have quite a lot of needles, some on my liver points, and they go in different places each week. My total is thirteen, and my dream is to beat my own record,' he says, with typical schoolboy relish.

He is unlikely to realize it. Oliver is now back to normal. His inhaler, which he used twice, has been mislaid, and he is able to sleep at nights without being disturbed by fits of coughing. The cough has gone, and he is attending every two months just so that the doctor can keep an eye on his progress.

Colitis

Nothing seemed to help Peter W.'s colitis. In a year of treatment with steroids to help the coating of the bowel, others which went into the bloodstream, and a foam which he had to inject into his rectum, he was still rushing to the lavatory every half hour, constantly passing blood, unable to sleep and losing weight.

Eventually, the treatment made him impotent. 'This was a side-effect which the doctors told me they didn't think of mentioning. They also said they were relatively new pills, and they weren't quite sure what effects they might have. At that point, I decided there must be a better way, and I contacted a TCM doctor I had seen on a television programme.'

The doctor found a lot of inflammation in the guts caused by damp, heat and toxins which had to be cleared from the system. He gave the patient two lots of pills, tiny things that looked like shotgun pellets. Mr W. had to take ten of one type, and twenty of the other every day. 'Dr Ke said the pills were to toughen up the bowel, and that's exactly how it feels. He told me it might take two years to cure me, and I think it was a couple of months before I knew definitely that I was on the mend.'

Treatment centred on the kidney, which is responsible for the antibodies which protect the system from disease. One of these forms a lining in the gut, and when this is damaged, colitis is the result. Before starting to work on the kidney, however, the doctor gave herbs to clean the body. 'We have a saying in TCM that even the best artist cannot paint a good picture without a clean white sheet of paper. One lot of medicine was to clear the toxins, the other was to treat the kidney.' The herbs included dandelion, rhubarb and ginseng.

Mr W. admitted, 'To be honest, I was sceptical at first. Only desperation took me there. When I first felt an improvement, I thought I was imagining it. I didn't want to give myself false hope. But as the weeks went by, I could see a marked improvement. I was impotent for two months after I came off the steroids, so they were obviously still in my system for that length of time.'

'I have been treated for just over a year, and the last time I saw the doctor, he told me that the new pills he was giving me would actually make me feel worse. He said they were to clear the infection from my body. He was right. I sometimes miss a day, and I feel better, but I am going to persist, because in my experience when he tells me something like that, I can rely on it.'

'I am now gaining weight, in fact I am having to watch what I eat. When my boys play football in the garden, I can kick the ball around with them now. Before, I didn't have the energy; even if I tried, I'd have to stop and hurry to the loo. If I hadn't tried TCM, I'm certain I wouldn't be playing football today.'

Colitis is one of the conditions which Western medicine finds difficult to treat. Surgery is often the final resort. TCM has a good success rate using herbal medicine.

Dermatitis

In the fifty years that he suffered from skin problems, Peter M. was never sure what the true nature of his illness was. It began when, as a young aircraft engineer during the war, he suffered a bad reaction after ethylene glycol leaked from a radiator and covered his hands and arms. A red, weeping rash spread down his arms and chest to his lower body, and he was treated for a time at the hospital in RAF Cranwell.

That was to be the first of many hospital stays in the years that followed. 'Every doctor seemed to call my skin condition by a different name. Dermatitis, eczema, other things. I never knew what it was. The irritation was terrible and eventually I was sent to a specialist skin hospital, where they did patch tests and discovered that I was reacting to quite a number of things but particularly to UV rays.'

Steroid creams controlled the condition to some degree, but a very acute attack soon followed, where his skin was so badly affected that he was swathed in dressings and wore special gloves. Steroid tablets brought some relief, but when he was weaned off them, the problem came back. At seventy-one years of age, Mr M. was reluctant to continue on steroids, and went to the TCM clinic near his home 'as a complete sceptic, but out of desperation'.

One of the top consultants from the Skin Disease Research Institute at Changzheng Hospital in Tianjin was on secondment to the Bath Clinic. Dr Liu has published several papers on the treatment of dermatitis erythematosa, eczema, lupus and psoriasis, and she explained through an interpreter that a skin disease as longstanding as Peter's would take many months to cure.

Peter was treated for six months before the skin began to heal. 'But on the other hand, it never got any worse either, and after what I had gone through before, that was a bonus in itself.'

Thereafter, the improvement started and within weeks his skin was absolutely clear. It stayed that way for seven months, then came a minor relapse. 'It is only on my scalp, neck and hands this time, but nothing like it used to be. It's more inconvenient and embarrassing than painful, and although I haven't started to recover yet, it is not getting any worse. This is my second month of treatment, and I will keep on taking it.

'I don't know if Dr Liu was surprised or disappointed to see me back again. She gives me lovely smiles, and we're great friends, but of course we can't converse, so I don't really know what her opinion is about this recurrence.'

Epilepsy

The first indication of David B.'s illness came when he was a small baby. Although he was a contented child, he would have spasms of going rigid and staring fixedly ahead. His parents thought this must be some form of infantile temper tantrum. The thought that he might be having some kind of fit did not cross their minds.

The episodes receded as he grew, but returned at adolescence, increasing in frequency and severity. Eventually, he was having three attacks every week, often injuring himself and others in the process.

'I'm not a violent person, but I used to break doors down and I've kicked people during a fit. I've injured myself scores of times, and the fits themselves used to drain me to such an extent that I had to spend the following day in bed, recovering.'

When he had an attack in the street, passers-by inevitably assumed he was drunk, and left him lying. His family started putting notes in his pockets giving his address, explaining that he was epileptic and asking people to help him.

Conventional drugs did control the fits to some degree, but did not allow him anything like a normal life. He appeared to be in a permanent trance, and his mother's anxiety increased. 'He seemed to be turning into a zombie and I felt he was literally fading away under my eyes.'

When doctors suggested increasing the dose, Mr B.'s mother told them that she felt it was exchanging one illness for another. 'What is the point of a life spent in a permanently drugged condition where my son hardly knows where he is?' she asked. By this time, though a mature adult in his late thirties, he was scarcely able to take such decisions himself.

In desperation, his mother took her son to visit a TCM doctor, who said that the treatment would take some time, but he was hopeful that he might be able to improve Mr B.'s condition. The herbal treatment took the form of tiny pills, and he was put on a strict diet: no sweet things, nothing fried, no dairy products except for a small amount of skimmed milk, and no alcohol.

The family noticed an improvement in Mr B. within the first two weeks of treatment. 'He was brighter and more alert, and as the weeks went on his condition got better and better. You couldn't recognize him as the same man, he was so dramatically improved.'

Once his condition stabilized, Mr B. was able to decrease the number of orthodox drugs he had continued to take throughout his TCM treatment. He is still taking one pill per day prescribed by his own GP.

'I am very well. I no longer feel moody or depressed and lead a normal life. Before that, I was a misery to myself and everyone around me.'

Eight-year-old Gemma's problems began with headaches, then sickness, and eventually she began walking around in an abnormal dream-like state, while her general health seemed to deteriorate rapidly. The family doctor thought the child's condition required further investigation and sent her to hospital in Oxford to have a brain scan.

Her mother was already attending a TCM doctor, and she mentioned the little girl's problem when she was having treatment. 'He told me to bring her in for an examination. Then he told me that she had severe epilepsy. Days later, I returned to the hospital for the results of the scan, and they diagnosed the same thing. They wanted to put her on a special drug, and predicted that she would start to have attacks twice daily.

'I told them a TCM doctor had already diagnosed epilepsy, through his pulse and tongue examination, and that I would try Gemma on herbal medicine first. The specialist said she really ought to take the drug they prescribed, and warned again about the frequency of the fits she would have without it.

'She has been having herbal medicine for five years, and she has never had a fit. The TCM doctor has her on a strict diet – she hasn't to eat chocolate, or any convenience foods like burgers, which is difficult for a teenager among all her friends. I know she cheats, and so does the doctor, but he is controlling her condition in spite of that. Nobody who didn't know her medical history would realize there was anything wrong with her, she's just a normal, healthy teenager.

'If it hadn't been for TCM treatment, I am sure she would have been on heavy medication all this time.'

Granula anularis

Two red spots resembling insect bites were the first symptoms which Mrs P. noticed. She assumed that she had been bitten, and was not unduly concerned despite the fact that the spots looked very angry, and caused what she recalls was 'the most excruciating itch', not just on the legs but also her arms, after she took a shower.

She mentioned it to her doctor, but he did not make any comment. 'Unsurprisingly, really, because I am one of those unfortunate people who get a lot of allergies. I suffer from asthma, hay fever and bronchitis. Also, I didn't actually mention the spots, just the itching in my limbs.'

When the spots cleared later, they left red circles with a brown centre, and this time the GP referred his patient to a consultant who sent samples of tissue for a biopsy. Granula anularis was diagnosed. 'I was told was that it was unusual in someone of my age. The doctor said it would resolve itself eventually, but could take months or years. There is a treatment which involves massive doses of vitamins or drugs to thin the blood, and having been a nurse I wasn't too keen to take anything like that.'

By the time Mrs P. consulted a TCM dermatologist, the condition affected the inner side of her thighs and calves. The itch was particularly bad and affected her sleep. 'Dr Liu prescribed herbal teas which I took night and morning, and the first night I took them I enjoyed the first calm, uninterrupted sleep I'd had for two years. The dosage was varied as I progressed and within months it had gone.

'There's no proof that the herbal medicine cured me, since the condition is supposed to clear up eventually, and it is not impossible that this is what happened. All I can say from my personal experience is that from the day I started to take it, I immediately felt so much better, that I could not believe the improvement. I am sure it was the herbal treatment which cured it.'

Guillian Barre Syndrome

This is an auto-immune disease, in which the peripheral nerves are destroyed. It is a relatively rare condition, first identified during the First World War. It affects about 1,000 people in Britain every year. It often follows a virus infection. Although some new forms of treatment are showing promise, there is no positive treatment so far, apart from steroids. Fortunately, in two-thirds of cases, particularly in young victims, the body heals itself again within three to six months.

In Barbara C.'s case, the virus struck after a bout of flu, and she began to notice that her legs and feet were beginning to go numb. Within two weeks she was paralysed from the waist down. She could not feel her legs at all, and suffered bad pain in her lower back. She was rushed into the Intensive Care Unit of the local hospital, and then transferred to the neuro-surgical ward for tests to see if the trouble stemmed from the spine. It was then that Guillian Barre Syndrome was diagnosed.

Doctors told her that the condition might cure itself, but also warned that if there was no improvement within a couple of years, she might be among the one-third of sufferers who do not recover, or take many years to do so. After a year in which there was no progress, she was taken off the steroid treatment, despite being still in a lot of pain.

Mrs C. was recommended to try TCM acupuncture by a friend who had undergone successful treatment for multiple sclerosis. 'The disease started when I was fifty-three, so the outlook didn't look very promising in my case. I don't know if it was the acupuncture which helped me or not, as this is such an unpredictable disease. All I can say is that as soon as I had the first session, I immediately felt the effects of pain relief, and slowly after that, my condition began to improve. I started to get the feeling back in my legs. My hands and arms, which had also been affected, are now back to normal.

'I am not yet 100 per cent fit. My feet go numb by the end of the day, but in the last six months I have improved immensely. I had been ill for a year when I first consulted Connie, and now, two years later, I feel wonderful. I have treatment every month or six weeks now, and my arthritis, which I also suffered from, is also much better.

'I was on painkillers for the first eighteen months of my illness, but after I began having acupuncture I was able to stop taking them.'

Hay fever

At the age of twelve, Mary C. developed hay fever, and for the following fifteen years, each summer became a nightmare of discomfort. She was often unable to leave the house, and lost weeks of schooling.

Anti-histamine injections stopped her nose running but did not clear the blocked tubes, and caused her face to swell. 'It seemed that every treatment which cut down on one of the symptoms produced side-effects which were just as bad,' she recalls.

At the first sight of flowers, she would develop a high temperature, swollen eyes, a streaming nose and intense pressure in the sinuses. 'I blew my nose so much that I had frequent nosebleeds. I had my nose cauterized several times, but it still didn't help.'

An advertisement in the local paper led her to seek help from a TCM doctor. 'I had tried herbal treatment, homoeopathy, and I'd spent a fortune at the chemist's, but I was still no nearer finding a cure.' She was given a bag of herbs to boil each morning and drink twice daily. After three days, she went back for a check-up. 'I can't describe how foul the medicine was. The doctors warned me it would taste bitter, and said that unless I was prepared to persevere with it, they couldn't help me.

'When I tasted that initial mouthful, I literally staggered back, it was so frightful, but I knew I had to face it, so I decided to sit down and wait for it to cool, and then try to down it in one go. While I was waiting, I literally felt the pressure easing from my face. That was what spurred me on. I knew that something was happening, and I was prepared to take anything that would get rid of my hay fever. The good thing is, there's no aftertaste, so if you can bring yourself to swallow it, the ordeal is over.'

Miss C.'s prescription was adjusted at her second visit, and this did not work so well. It also made her sick. The third change, however, led to an even greater improvement. After the fourth course of herbs, the doctor told her she was cured.

Treatment took two weeks.

Infertility

The prospect of ever becoming a father began to look depressingly remote when Richard S. was told the reason behind his partner's inability to conceive. They had waited over a year before seeking a medical opinion, and now tests showed that his body was producing antibodies which were attacking his own semen. 'In other words,' he recalls, 'every sperm I produced came equipped with its own home-made condom.'

Treatment for this form of infertility involves high doses of steroids for long periods of time. There was also a small chance that IVF might be successful, if the sperm was 'washed' before being introduced to the egg.

As an osteopath, Mr S. was unwilling to start on steroid therapy, and sufficiently open-minded to consider other means of treatment. He made inquiries at a TCM clinic and was told that one of the doctors there had treated several similar cases in his hospital in China.

Dr Chen's prognosis at Mr S.'s first examination was that there was a 60–70 per cent chance of success within a year. In this instance, the tea from the large bag of herbs was not particularly bad to take, and only had to be swallowed once daily. Three months later, Richard's partner was pregnant.

The consultant at the IVF unit of the local hospital knew about the TCM treatment, and responded positively to Mr S.'s suggestion that they carry out a second sperm test. It showed that the condition was unchanged, or if anything slightly worse than the last time.

'I tried to discuss this with the TCM doctor, but the language problem is a barrier as we have to talk through an interpreter, and so I don't know whether the treatment worked or not. It seems to me that there are three possible explanations.

'First, that it succeeded by some other means without destroying the antibodies, though I find that possibility difficult to accept; second, as there was a gap of over a month between the pregnancy and my second sperm test, that my sperm changed when I was taking the herbs, but reverted back again as soon as I stopped; or third, as does happen on rare occasions, that it was sheer chance that one unaffected sperm got through.

'The doctor told me that papers on the efficacy of the treatment had been produced in China, and I would love to be able to get hold of them, to read the data. If Chinese research papers were available here, we might get some insight into the infertility work they are doing, and it would help towards a better understanding of the treatment.'

Dr Chen's examination revealed a deficiency of both yin and yang in the kidneys and he prescribed herbs which would nourish both, and also strengthen the back and the spleen. The herbs included epimedium, to tonify the kidney, strengthen yang, dispel the wind and eliminate dampness. Prepared rehmannia root, which is mixed with yellow rice, amomun fruit and tangerine peel and then dried in the sun, was given to nourish the blood, tonify yin and replenish the vital essence and the marrow.

Leg ulcers

Miss W. already had a problem with varicose veins in her legs before the ulcers started. She thought she was developing varicose eczema, and as she had always had a preference for complementary medicine, she decided to consult a Chinese doctor whose name she got from a local health shop.

'By the time two ulcers developed on each side of my leg, just above the ankle, I was in considerable pain. The doctor gave me an oil which he told me had sixty-eight different herbs in it, as well as prescribing medicine, and now, after a year's treatment, all that remains of the larger ulcer is one tiny hole. The other has healed up completely.'

The doctor's first step was to treat Miss W.'s overall condition. Her blood vessels were at fault in his view, and he gave herbs which would improve the quality of the blood itself. He included the famous dan gui (angelica root), well known for its ability to improve the blood, plus safflower, peach kernel and astragalus, all of which would also strengthen the spleen and liver. The herbs would help the organs to move the blood and make it less sticky.

'I still see the doctor every six weeks, and he has been treating me for the terrible headaches I get as a result of cervical spondylitis, which I also suffer from. My GP had me on Brufin tablets, but I don't like taking heavy drugs. When I mentioned the headaches to the TCM doctor, he explained that the blood vessels were constricted so the blood was not reaching the brain properly, and the pain stemmed from the blood trying to force its way up into the head. He said he could prescribe medicine to help the circulation. Since I got the Chinese herbs, I have weaned myself off the painkillers, and I haven't had a headache.'

Myalgic encephalomyelitis (ME)

When doctors told Julian C. that he had bone cancer, he was shocked, but not surprised. He felt so weak and ill that the diagnosis seemed inevitable.

Then, following further tests, he was informed that there was no evidence of any malignancy. None of the consultants could say precisely what the trouble was. One doctor suggested it was psychosomatic and prescribed tranquillizers. 'I knew that my illness was certainly not in my mind and refused to take them.' Further tests followed, after which a haemotologist diagnosed a form of ME.

Mr C.'s medical problems began in his late thirties after a bout of glandular fever. Until then, he had been a keen marathon runner with a strong and vigorous constitution.

Now, every joint in his body ached, he had constant headaches, permanent lethargy, and – though he managed to continue working throughout the three years of his illness – he had to change to afternoon shifts, because in the mornings he was physically unable to get out of bed.

He tried TCM on the recommendation of his father-in-law who had been treated for a skin complaint. 'The doctor looked at my tongue and read my pulse, and told me that my qi was very weak and that my liver was full of toxins. He said that within ten days of taking the medicine I would feel better, within three weeks I would feel well, and within three months I wouldn't need to see him anymore. Then he gave me the bag full of road sweepings, as we called it, and I came home and started to take them.'

The doctor's prognosis was wrong. Mr C.'s improvement started well before ten days. Before the week was out, the aches that had plagued him for years had disappeared, and the headaches had eased. He returned the following week, the herbal mixture was adjusted, and within the fortnight he began to feel his energy returning.

'As the weeks went by, I started to see the difference in my tongue. It had been coated with white fur, swollen and blotchy and very sore. Now it started to regain a healthy pink colour. All my energy returned, and after seven visits to the doctor, he told me that, unless I wanted it, there was no reason for me to go back. I was cured. That was a year ago, and I haven't had a problem since. I am running again, and I feel great.

'After my recovery, I met one of the doctors who had treated me, and told him about my treatment. He said it was obviously the placebo effect, and that was that. I wrote to one consultant who diagnosed ME, because he had been very good and took a great interest in my case. He had told me to take life as easy as possible, get as much rest as I could, and that it would eventually go away.

'I wrote to him afterwards, thinking he would want to know about my cure, in case it could help patients with the same problem. He never acknowledged my letter.'

Motor neurone disease

When John M. was diagnosed as suffering from motor neurone disease his daughter, an occupational therapist, began searching for treatments which might arrest the progress of the disease. She suggested her father should try TCM treatment, and take evening primrose oil, about which she had read encouraging reports in scientific journals.

Mr M. consulted an acupuncture expert at a Chinese medical clinic, at a point where he had suffered slow loss of muscular strength and control of movement, accompanied by muscular atrophy. He was unable to tie up his shoelaces, and could not pick up small items such as a sheet of paper or a safety pin.

'At my first session, Professor Wang told me he thought Chinese acupuncture could help to stabilize the condition in about a year, and that thereafter I might become well enough to stop the treatment altogether, and then I could be monitored regularly and have acupuncture only if and when it was needed.

'There's an idea that acupuncture isn't painful, but in my case it certainly is. I have needles placed all the way down my spine – over twenty each time – they are inserted very deeply and they do hurt. For an hour or so afterwards I can feel decidedly groggy. I usually find, however, that after a session my limp disappears for a day or so.'

Mr M. is not convinced that his MND has been stabilized and, in measuring his own progress, thinks there has been a slight deterioration over recent months. Unfortunately, he caught flu in the winter epidemic, and this proved a great setback, as Dr Wang had predicted. Before that, he had noticed a definite improvement. After eleven treatments, the movement in his arm increased and he was once more able to tie laces and grasp small objects between his finger and thumb, movements which he had not been able to achieve in the past two years.

'When MND was confirmed by specialists, I asked them to be blunt, and they were. I was told 1 would lose weight as my muscles wasted, and although I lost half a stone when I had flu, I have regained all but two pounds, and I am still gaining.

'I can't be certain any of this is attributable to TCM. I am also taking large doses of evening primrose oil, and I feel that has been helpful in the weight gain. I told my GP of the other medicines I was trying, and he told me acupuncture wouldn't help but evening primrose might. He also wrote to the hospital when I started acupuncture, to ask if the consultant would wish to monitor my progress, but he wasn't interested.

'Motor neurone disease is an unpredictable condition, which varies from person to person, and it is therefore difficult to draw any reliable conclusions from one's own experience. All I know is that I have faith in Dr Wang, and I find I can rely on what he tells me.

'Occasionally after my weekly session he will say that I won't feel any effects for three days, and that is always the case. He still assures me that he can control the condition and that 1 may be able to come off treatment for good once that point is reached. Since I started acupuncture, I certainly have more energy, and feel more optimistic.

'However, I must be cautious. I do detect signs of deterioration, and I know my disease is still there. I certainly feel that TCM has been helpful, but how much my improvement is due to acupuncture and how much to evening primrose oil is difficult to tell.'

Multiple sclerosis (herbal treatment)

Shortly after the birth of her first baby, Joan R. was diagnosed as suffering from multiple sclerosis, the degenerative disease of the central nervous system caused by damage to the myolin sheath which protects the nerve fibres. The cause is unknown, and affects women more often than men. In some cases, the disease only attacks once, but the usual pattern follows a course of attacks and remissions. Symptoms include problems with weakness, numbness and lack of co-ordination, blurred vision, poor memory and kidney dysfunction.

After the first five years, the MS went into remission, and the patient had no further attacks for fifteen years. Then the disease became active again, and as well as suffering loss of mobility Mrs R. became prone to constant chest infections and repeated bouts of cystitis.

The episodes were so frequent and prolonged that eventually she began to develop an immunity to most of the antibiotics she constantly had to take. Her bladder problems were so severe that she became incontinent. She was referred to hospital for tests to check for kidney damage, but decided instead to take the advice of a woman living in the same village, and seek treatment from a Chinese medicine clinic.

Her treatment involved a weekly visit to the clinic, where she was diagnosed as suffering from a deficiency of the qi of the kidney yang, and excess heat in the lung and the bladder. She was given a mixture of herbs which she had to prepare at home, and drink each day. Included in the prescription was mulberry mistletoe and Scutellaria root to dry up dampness in the body. Within a couple of months of starting treatment, she began to feel much better. 'I had more energy, the pain lessened, and my urine infections cleared up almost completely.

'I began to get a general feeling of well-being, and the depression I had been prone to also lifted as I started to improve. I have had a couple of bouts of cystitis in the year since I started treatment, but they have been short-lived and have cleared up of their own accord.'

When, later, her appointment came through from the hospital, she duly had the kidney x-rays, which showed that there was no damage or sign of infection. In view of her past medical history, the doctors were naturally surprised, and Mrs R. told them of the herbal medicine she was taking.

'They were non-committal and said it obviously wasn't doing me any harm, but my GP thinks my improvement is just a placebo effect. My own view is that TCM has been extremely helpful. I still attend every fortnight, and my prescription includes extra herbs which help to keep me going. The doctor says that my progress is being maintained, and he is pleased with the way things are progressing.

'The medicine changes regularly – I can recognize the herbs now. There are usually about sixteen ingredients, and the doctor will add or take away some according to my condition. The medicine tastes like liquid tar. Truly awful, but I am becoming used to it.

'In the winter, the whole family came down with flu, but I sailed through without so much as a cold. Before I started taking the herbs, I had prolonged and frequent chest infections and fevers and got everything that was going. I know that TCM can't cure MS, but it does deal with the attendant ailments very effectively, and I feel like a different person.

'I'm more optimistic, I have more energy, and I can cope with my condition. Five years ago, a hospital consultant told me they would find the cure for MS within a couple of years, and nothing has happened so far. I'm sure that they will come up with a remedy before too long, and that thought, together with the TCM treatment, is what keeps me going.'

Multiple sclerosis (acupuncture)

Because she had so many other complaints which her China-trained acupuncturist was treating, Doreen B. never mentioned the blindness in her left eye, caused by optic neuritis. Although she believes that MS developed after the birth of her first child, the disease was not diagnosed until years later, and took a slow but steady grip on her body in the first fifteen years after her GP broke the news about her illness.

'At first, I suspected I had a brain tumour, as I had lost vision in one eye, I had no balance, and I had attacks when I couldn't move at all, so the knowledge that I had MS actually came as a relief,' she remembers. When, five years ago, Doreen began treatment with Connie, who had studied TCM acupuncture in Nanjing, she had also developed rheumatoid arthritis and osteoporosis, and had a problem involving the sacrum, the bone at the base of the spinal column, which doctors said stemmed from an injury sustained during childbirth.

'I was in such pain and had so much wrong with me that I never even thought about my eye,' she said. 'Connie told me that she couldn't cure my arthritis, but she could relieve it, and she has certainly done that. The needles seem to take the inflammation away, and the effect lasts for one to two weeks before it wears off. As far as the MS goes, my condition has not regressed at all since I started treatment, and I have not had any bladder problems since.

'Frequency of urination is another complication of the disease, and I suffered badly with that, but after the first four or five treatments, I never had any more bother.

'I still have a bowel retention problem, but I see Connie every fortnight, and she puts me right again. I also take Ephamol, the high-dosage evening primrose oil, and I believe that has been a great help too. I can't speak too highly of the difference acupuncture has made to my life.

'Most amazingly, a couple of years ago, I started to get vision back in my eye. All I could see was dark and light to begin with, then slowly it cleared and I saw colours again. My vision isn't perfect, I can't make out small details, but I can see reasonably well.

'I feel so much better. My depression has gone, my balance is back, I can climb up three flights of stairs unaided, whereas before I could hardly walk. I am very lucky in that I have the most marvellous support from my orthodox consultants. I see a neurologist and a rheumatologist, and they both know I have Chinese acupuncture, and both urge me to go on with it, because they say it is doing me so much good.

'I should be on six different types of tablet daily, but in fact I only take one pill for my rheumatoid arthritis, and one painkiller. For the rest, my acupuncture treatment keeps me well. There are times when I will have some crisis, but when that happens I ring Connie and go for a treatment as soon as she can fit me in.

'Last week I got optic neuritis in my right eye. The pain and swelling were awful, but one session with the needles and it went back to normal within days.'

Muscular dystrophy

A family friend persuaded nine-year-old Gary's parents to take him to the doctor. She felt he needed attention for his mouth, which 'didn't move properly'. When he was a baby, the boy had fallen from a chair, hurting his face quite badly and putting his teeth through his lip. His parents assumed that this is what had caused the problem.

They were shocked to learn that their son had muscular dystrophy. 'Especially when doctors said nothing could be done for him. We would have to live with it, and hope that a cure was found before he grew up.'

The boy was twenty-one before the family learned of a Chinese doctor practising nearby. When Gary went to see him, the doctor said that his chest had become so concave that within five years it would crush his heart and lungs.

His treatment consists of acupuncture and herbal medicine, and in two years his mother says the effect has been gradual, but marked. 'Gary's chest muscles have grown and other muscles are now beginning to grow. He still hasn't got any strength, but the doctor says that will come last of all. He has to concentrate on building up his body first.

'If my son fell over, he couldn't get up unaided, but he knows within himself how much better he feels, and how different he is. The herbs he takes are terrible to taste, but he sits there as the rest of the family has tea, laughing as he drinks them down and telling us he's having the best drink of the day. The doctor is confident that he'll build him up and cure him, and I am equally sure that, with time, he will.'

Prostate

When sixty-year-old John B.'s bladder problems began, the deterioration followed rapidly over the next six months. 'I couldn't have a drink of water without having to rush to pass water half an hour afterwards. My GP sent me to see a specialist, and he said, 'No problem, a minor operation will soon put that to rights,' but I didn't like the idea of surgery, so I decided to consult a Chinese doctor to see if there was any prospect of treatment without involving surgery.

'That was nine months ago. I have been on herbal tablets since and although I am still aware that I am not back to normal, I am very much better. The TCM doctor told me the problem stemmed from a kidney weakness, and that he would work on that, and on my general state of health, because I also had a problem with asthma. I now go every three months, and the doctor told me that the last lot of medicine he gave me should also help to ease that problem.

'My asthma hasn't troubled me since then, but coincidentally I also decided to get a cleaner to do the house at the same time. I know the asthma is aggravated by dust, and as I'm a bachelor, and not very good about housework, I suppose I don't help myself. So whether it is the medicine, or the effects of less dust about the place, I really can't say.'

The doctor's treatment concentrated on the kidneys, because once they were strengthened, the quality of the urine would improve, and the condition would clear itself. Because the kidney was not working properly, poor urine was irritating the prostate gland. The kidneys, in TCM, are responsible for 'inhaling' the air. The lungs exhale and govern the breathing, but the kidneys 'grasp' the incoming breath to help the lungs and retain it in the body. When older people have problems with breathing, it is considered to be because the kidneys are becoming tired and not inhaling efficiently.

Treatment for breathing conditions usually involves the kidney, and the herbs the doctor prescribed are also used in the treatment of asthma. John's new domestic routine would certainly help, smiled the doctor, but it was the herbs that really did the trick.

Psoriasis

Chinese medicine was a last resort for Oliver H. In twenty years as a psoriasis victim he had tried every type of therapy from modern medicine to cold tar baths, with very little response. Only the sun seemed to clear his skin, and that was a very temporary effect. When he consulted Dr Liu, he had large red lesions all over his face and body, the skin was painful and itchy and he was unable to sleep. His pulse was wiry and slippery, and his tongue was very red. The doctor prescribed herbal granules to cool the blood and reduce heat and dampness in the liver and gallbladder meridian.

After one week on herbal granules, the colour of the infected skin was paler, the skin was less flaky, and Mr H. felt that his general health was also better. The improvement continued over the course of the year. In the early spring, there was a sudden flare-up, which the doctor said was due to a cold weather reaction. She used stronger medicine, containing ten herbs, to increase the cooling effect, and changed the evening prescription for one which would nourish the yin.

The morning medicine contained herbs which would reduce the dampness in Mr H.'s body, and cool the blood. The evening herbs had a similar effect, but opened another channel to reduce the dampness more effectively. The medicines contained scrophularia root, which nourishes the yin and reduces blood heat, plus honeysuckle and isatis leaf to reduce heat and toxins, and gentian root to cool the liver and gallbladder.

Three changes were made in the prescriptions over a course of two years, during which time the patient continued to improve. He went through the second winter of his treatment without a single outbreak. In the past, the psoriasis had always got worse during the cold weather.

Raynaud's disease and scleroderma

Raynaud's disease is named after the physician Maurice Raynaud who published his thesis, 'Gangrene and Intermittent Asphyxia of the Extremities', in 1862. It is a condition in which the blood supply, usually to the fingers and toes, but sometimes also to the ears and nose, is interrupted. It causes severe pain, numbness and tingling. In some sufferers, the condition may cause nothing more than minor discomfort, but in extreme cases it can lead to ulcers or even gangrene.

Scleroderma is a skin condition in which the hands and feet, and sometimes other parts of the body, become tough and leathery due to swelling and thickening of the porous tissues. Internal changes may also cause difficulty in swallowing, loss of weight, aching muscles, joints and bones, shortness of breath and kidney troubles.

The two conditions often go together, which happened in the case of Ann B., a state registered nurse who had suffered for eight years before beginning TCM treatment. She also developed Sjogren's syndrome, a condition where the body fails to produce saliva or tears, and this in turn led to lymphoma, requiring radiotherapy treatment.

Despite her deteriorating health, Mrs B. is, by her own description, a determined and positive person who did not allow her physical state to affect her mental attitude. She was supported by a caring and dedicated doctor at London's Royal Free Hospital, who had tried several Western treatments on the patient, with limited success. A variety of complementary treatments proved similarly disappointing.

A relative who had TCM treatment for ME urged her to try herbal medicine, and Mrs B. agreed to one last experience of alternative therapy. 'I was in a very low state by this time. It was such an effort to peel a potato that it took hours to prepare dinner. At bedtime, I crawled upstairs on all-fours. I decided that if I was going to try Chinese medicine, I would persist with the treatment for a year, to give it a chance to work.

'At my first consultation, I mentioned the mouth ulcers which I had suffered from for years. To my surprise, the doctor insisted on treating them first. He explained that they were the result of too much heat, whereas my other complaints arose from heat deficiency, and would require different treatment. Almost immediately, the ulcers cleared up and I have never had one since.' Dr Chen diagnosed weakness of qi and blood with deficiency of yang, stagnation of qi and blood with excess heat in the upper burner.

His treatment was intended to produce more yang and qi, nourish the blood, assist the qi circulation and reduce the stagnation.

For the following nine months, the patient prepared and drank herbs twice daily, eating no food for an hour before or after taking the medicine. Herbs included safflower (good for blood circulation and removing blood stasis) and Chinese angelica root, a herb that is particularly efficient at treating blood conditions, improving the circulation, relieving pain and regularizing the bowels. It is often prescribed for menstrual difficulties and is used as a tonic herb for women.

'Before my illness, I had played County League tennis, but all that had ended. Two months after my herbal treatment began, I started to feel better. Within four months I was back on court, able to hit the ball – admittedly without any power behind it. By six months, however, I could run around the court and put some force behind my serve. My friends were absolutely astonished.'

Mrs B. continues to take the anti-inflammatory drugs, the drops and the mouth spray which were prescribed by the hospital, but she no longer needs painkillers.

'The pain used to be absolutely excruciating. Now, I feel so much better it's difficult to explain. My eyes are alive again. Before, they looked lifeless. I am in control of myself again. The doctor is optimistic that he can cure me completely, and I hope that before long I will be able to do without treatment.

'I was treated weekly for the first three months, then monthly, and now, a year later, the doctor feels I have almost reached the point when I can stop. I still feel I have a little way to go, but there is no doubt about the extent of my improvement.'

Rheumatoid arthritis

No birthday present was ever more unwelcome than the one which greeted Rae L. on her fortieth birthday. She developed rheumatoid arthritis, and for the following three years was in a steady decline, taking anti-inflammatory drugs which, in the first instance, didn't have any effect. Her doctor changed the tablets, but the second lot, she felt, made her condition worse. 'I stopped taking them, so perhaps you could say I never gave them a chance. I decided to try acupuncture instead.

'That immediately helped with the pain, and to a limited extent it treated the arthritis too, but after a while we reached stalemate. The acupuncturist was a student of a TCM doctor. He felt he couldn't do any more for me, but thought his teacher could, so I made an appointment to see him.

'Dr Ke told me from the outset that he couldn't cure my condition, but that he could make life a lot better for me. That was a year ago, and I am not just better, but incredibly better. Before the treatment, I could only just walk, using sticks, but it was extremely painful. The condition was worst in my legs, but it was also in my shoulders and my arms.

'Within weeks of taking the herbs, I was able to ride a bike. My shoulders are much better, and I can now do little jobs like turning taps on, which were impossible before. I still have aches in my wrists, knees and ankles, but they are definitely improving, and although I still walk slowly I can go into town on a shopping trip without any ill effects. Shopping used to be a nightmare.

'Rheumatoid arthritis is extremely painful. The ache is in the joints, the muscles and the ligaments, but it also makes you feel generally ill. Now I feel well again, in all-round good health. The doctor told me that it would take a long time to get results, but I feel it has been very quick. My joints are not so swollen, and my knees actually look like knees again, whereas before they were quite unrecognizable. The heat has gone out of them.

'I also had very bad period pains all my life. Before my children were born, I used to have to spend the first day in bed. On my initial consultation with the TCM doctor, he took a full medical history, and asked a lot of other questions such as whether I was a worrier, and if I felt the cold badly. I mentioned my period problems, he gave me herbs for that, and I haven't had a pain since.

'I still see a rheumatologist, despite the fact that I have declined all the tablets he has offered me. I told him I was going to try Chinese medicine, and he was very sceptical. He thought it was cranky, but he took the view that what I did was up to me. He has kept an eye on my progress and he is delighted with my improvement. I used to go every six months, but he only wants to see me once a year now.'

A TCM doctor looks to see what is going wrong with the body when every joint is swollen. His examination aims to find out the cause. In Rae's case, the whole immune system had broken down. There were dampness and heat in her body, which had to be cleared.

The reason he was unable to cure the patient was because once the joints are damaged, this is irreversible. If the condition is caught in the early stages, herbs will rebalance the body, and there is a very good chance of a complete cure.

Slipped disc

As an active, busy wife and mother whose hobby was weight-training, Emma B. found it particularly hard to take when she developed a back problem which the doctor diagnosed as a slipped disc. The pain was intense, she had no strength in her legs, movement of any kind was agony, and all that she had to help the condition were strong painkillers and anti-inflammatory drugs. They helped to alleviate the pain, but not to remove it.

Mrs B. went for private treatment to an osteopath three times a week, but he told her that he thought a small piece of disc had actually snapped off, and he could not help. He suggested that she ask for a hospital appointment, because surgery might be the only answer.

Mrs B.'s husband was working at the home of a TCM doctor at the time, and mentioned his wife's problem. Dr Lee said he thought acupuncture would help, and when she had a consultation, he diagnosed a blood clot trapped in a nerve in the spine. She was given acupuncture treatment and herbal medicine. 'I was able to come off the drugs immediately. The doctor didn't want me to take them because he said they would impair the rest of my system, and I was hesitant about giving them up, but the first treatment made me feel so much better, I no longer needed them.'

Although the pain went very quickly, the weakness in Mrs B.'s legs remained and the doctor told her that he needed to work to stabilize her condition. It took several more sessions before she was able to exert enough force on the clutch to enable her to drive the car, but after a year of weekly treatment, the pain was gone, her strength had returned, and she was living an active life once more.

Since then, her entire family has had TCM treatment, with very positive results. She says she never sees her GP now. 'I have such faith in my TCM doctor that I go to him first. I know my case was very complicated, because I could only have an appointment once a week, when the doctor's assistant was there to help him. He needed someone on hand while he worked, and I remember one day, as he was putting the needles in, he remarked to the assistant that in the wrong hands, the technique he was using could cause paralysis.

'That gave me a moment's unease, but I know how competent and experienced he is, and I have utter faith in him. He cured me completely, and I have never looked back.'

Thyroid

When Mrs R. discovered a lump in her throat, she suspected that the problem might be cancer, and was naturally relieved to find, after hospital tests, that the problem was caused by two cysts which were pressing against the thyroid gland.

'Unfortunately, they told me there was no diet I could go on, and no medicine to cure me. I would have to go on Thyroxine for the rest of my life. I felt terribly ill, I could hardly swallow, and I felt constantly as if I was choking. I was also suffering from menopausal symptoms, so I was in a very low state. I happened to read a series of articles on Chinese medicine in a Sunday magazine, and I wondered if that might be the answer to my problem.

'I had a wonderfully supportive GP, who said that since conventional medicine couldn't help me, there would be no harm in asking about TCM, and she wrote to the Chinese doctor on my behalf. He replied that herbal medicine could help, and although his surgery was a long way from my home, I travelled to London for a consultation.'

The diagnosis showed a problem with the kidneys, which in TCM theory control the endocrine system. The depression felt was part of the hormonal problem, and the doctor's prescription was meant to fine-tune her system. The liver and spleen had to be balanced, as the liver was failing to process the used hormones and expel them from the body. There was liver stagnation and spleen deficiency, and the treatment involved very subtle use of herbs to ensure that the deficient organs grew in strength together. If the liver stagnation was moved too quickly, the spleen would not be able to cope, and vice versa.

'The doctor gave me herbal tea which I have to drink three times daily, and pills which I take twice a day. Since then, I have had a new lease of life. The cysts are slowly getting smaller, and I feel well again. They sometimes tend to get larger around about the time I would have had a period, but it only lasts for a day or two, and then they shrink again.

'My menopausal problems were distressing too. I used to get palpitations, and a strange feeling as if I was floating in mid-air, which was very disorientating. I got to the state where I was afraid to go out, in case I had an attack in the street, but the doctor prescribed herbal pills for that and it has now gone completely.

'The tea and pills change from time to time, and I go for a check-up every two months. My GP monitored my progress, and she thought the herbal medicine had been very good for me. She was interested to learn more about it, but tragically she was killed in an avalanche during a skiing holiday.'

The TCM doctor is confident that within another three months or so, the cysts will have disappeared and the condition will be cured.

CHAPTER SIX
New Drugs from Old

One morning in 1989, a pharmacist running a small pharmaceutical consultancy in Cambridge received a phone call from a London paediatrician. The two had been students together, and the doctor, a skin specialist at Great Ormond Street Hospital for Children in London, was ringing to discuss a situation which was puzzling him. 'Some of my most difficult eczema cases are being cured,' Dr David Atherton told his friend. 'That isn't usually a problem,' replied Dr Geoffrey Guy. 'Not usually,' the dermatologist agreed. 'Only it isn't me who's curing them.'

So begins the now familiar story of how Chinese herbal medicine emerged from the confines of London's Soho to attract the interest and (at least in terms of its expertise in treating certain skin conditions which respond poorly to allopathic medicine) the respect of Western doctors working in Britain.

Dr Atherton explained how a succession of long-term outpatients suddenly appeared at his clinic showing a dramatic improvement in their condition. Since the remedies at his disposal could not produce such impressive and immediate results, he asked what could possibly have brought about such a transformation. It transpired that the children's despairing parents had taken them to consult a woman doctor in London's Chinatown, working in a cramped little basement room beneath a small shop stacked high with sacks of strange and exotic dried plants and herbs.

The mixture Dr Ding Hui Luo weighed out for them filled a large paper bag, and looked just like something raked up from a woodland garden in winter. Twigs, leaves, shrivelled blossoms and a number of quite unidentifiable objects were contained within it. Patients were instructed to boil it for an hour and drink the liquid. The taste was appalling. The effect was miraculous.

Dr Atherton was so intrigued that he went to see the doctor, and asked if she would co-operate in clinical trials on more of his patients so that he could monitor the treatment. She agreed to do so, early indications were favourable, and the National Eczema Society decided to fund a two-year study into the treatment.

The object of the telephone call was to ask whether Dr Guy's pharmaceutical company might be interested in researching the properties of these herbs, to establish which were the active agents in the brew, and to see if a way could be found to make the medicine easier to take, more palatable, and more acceptable to the Western concept of a prescription. It would also have to pass the stringent standards of various boards and committees.

Concocting a standard medicine based on traditional herbal remedies was an extremely challenging task. Western pharmacology is accustomed to drugs which contain a single active agent. It identifies a disease by name, and treats all sufferers with the same remedy. If six people appear at morning surgery with eczema symptoms, they will all leave with the same advice and medicine.

A TCM doctor identifies diseases by syndrome, and makes a diagnosis based on the patient as an individual. The name he or she gives the complaint will differ according to which part of the body is affected and the state of the patient's general health. In TCM, eczema has many causes. It could stem from the lungs, the stomach, heart or blood. It might be caused by heat, damp heat or wind.

One patient will leave the surgery having learned he has a 'syndrome of wind and heat in the blood'. Another may be told he has a 'syndrome of damp heat'. The herbs prescribed would vary markedly in each case, as they will have a different job to do, and as many as fifteen might be used in each prescription. Moreover, as the patient's condition altered, herbs would be added or subtracted.

The research team decided that their task lay in trying to find a formula which would respect the traditional approach, while translating it into a more Western concept of drug therapy; something that had never been attempted before.

The first standard formula reduced the number of herbs to ten, and standardized the weights. It was produced in the form of a tea-bag, making the medicine easier to take, and much quicker and simpler to prepare. It was named Zemaphyte. Early results were encouraging, producing an improvement in 60 per cent of cases. Not quite as impressive as the Soho doctor's individual herbal concoctions, but, in terms of treatment for hitherto intractable eczema, a considerable step forward.

Tests continued at Great Ormond Street to investigate the longer-term response of children who had completed the first study. Thirty-seven children who had taken part in the first double-blind placebo controlled trial were given the opportunity to continue treatment. At the end of a year, eighteen showed a 90 per cent reduction in eczema activity sores, and five showed lesser degrees of improvement. Ten children withdrew due to lack of response, and a further four because of the taste of the medicine, or the difficulty in its preparation. Liver function abnormalities presented in two patients, but their eczema was so well controlled that they were able to stop the treatment, and within eight weeks the liver function was back to normal.

The Zemaphyte formula is now available in granule form, but is expensive to produce and, following the NHS prescribing restrictions, no longer available on prescription. Longer-term studies will be needed to investigate the relationship between the herbal medicine and liver toxicity, and to ascertain whether the herbs actually cure eczema or alleviate the condition temporarily.

The experiment has achieved one important breakthrough in Britain. It has alerted the medical profession to the possibilities of new treatments brought about by a study of some of the drugs which have been used in China for generations. Scientists in Hong Kong, Japan, the United States and Europe have been carrying out research into Chinese herbs for several years, particularly since the race to beat the AIDS virus began.

In the University of California in San Francisco, a purified protein named trichosanthin, extracted from a cucumber-like plant called the Chinese snake gourd, is undergoing clinical trials as a potential treatment for AIDS. It seems to have an even more effective action against the HIV virus than AZT. Tian Hua Fen, as it is called, has been used in herbal medicine since the days of the Han Dynasty, over 2,000 years ago.

An extract from qinghao (*Artemisia apiacea*) is an effective new drug in the treatment of pernicious and cerebral malaria. In cancer, combined methods of Western and TCM therapies have shown promise in prolonging life-span. Chinese herbs and acupuncture treatment can markedly reduce the side-effects of radium and chemotherapy, as many patients being treated by TCM doctors in Britain know from personal experience.

Legend has it that the famous doctor Hua Tuo (see page 198) learned about the curative qualities of the evergreen artemisia (*Artemisia capillaris Thunberg*) from a patient who was so sick and shrivelled that his friends called him Mr Cockroach. The man was yellow with jaundice and Hua Tuo told him that there was no cure for his disease. Months later, the doctor met the man on the street. He was not only alive, but in good health.

Mr Cockroach assured the doctor that the illness had cured itself, but Hua Tuo knew that was unlikely. Closer questioning revealed that, because he was so sick, the man had not been able to work and had to live on a plant he gathered at the roadside. He showed the doctor the plant, and Hua Tuo started using it to treat jaundice. Unfortunately, it didn't work. Deciding that perhaps the time of harvesting had something to do with its effectiveness, the doctor waited to pick it at the same time of year as Mr Cockroach had done. This time, the patients recovered. Whether the story is true or not, evergreen artemisia is still used for liver and gallbladder complaints, to promote bile production and as a general anti-viral herb.

At the Institute of Materia Medica in Beijing, scientists have succeeded in extracting a substance from the bark of a tree which has a positive influence on cancer cells, and offers future hope for millions of sufferers. The problem at present is that only a few thousandths of a gram can be obtained from every kilogram of bark. Modern biotechnology may be able to overcome this problem if it is able to produce larger amounts in cell cultures. Such things have been done before. The active compound in aspirin is a synthetically produced and improved component of willow bark. In the ninety years since it first appeared on the market, the world's most famous pain reliever has become so popular that all the willow trees on earth could not supply the demand.

Increasingly, Chinese scientists are collaborating with Western colleagues to close the gap between ancient medical wisdom and modern technical expertise. At the Institute in Beijing, 600 scientists are working on the development of new drugs to combat cardiovascular complaints and strokes, as well as cancer. All are major causes of death in China, as they are in the West. A thistle-like plant, *Carthamus tinctorius*, is producing hopeful results in clinical trials in cases of angina pectoris.

Even the humble liquorice plant, used by Chinese physicians for over 3,000 years, and one of their favourite components in prescriptions to treat liver disorders like hepatitis, jaundice, nausea and vomiting, has been shown by modern research to do precisely what the ancients had always claimed. It is a demulcent (soothing agent), a spasmolytic (countering the muscle spasms that cause colic and some bronchial disorders), an expectorant (increasing the production of sputum), an antitussive (suppressing coughing) and an anti-inflammatory and antiallergic substance, which makes it particularly useful in the treatment of asthma.

It can produce adrenocortical hormones and reduce blood fat, and is effective in the treatment of leukaemia. It appears to have anti-depressant properties too, and to act as a muscle relaxant. It is mildly laxative and may have detoxifying effects on poisons such as strychnine. Not only is it able to protect the liver, and to offer short-term relief of stomach ulcers, it also counters bacterial growth and plaque, and so helps to prevent dental decay.

Every herb in the pharmacopoeia has some legend attached to it. The story of how liquorice came to be used so frequently in herbal medicine tells of a doctor who left home to visit country patients, and did not return. Townspeople kept turning up at the house, asking for treatment, and the doctor's wife felt she could not send them away empty-handed. Knowing nothing about medicine, she ate a little of each herb to see how it tasted ... sour, bitter, pungent, salty and sweet. Most patients would prefer the sweet-tasting medicine, she decided, and handed liquorice out liberally, regardless of the complaint.

By the time the doctor came home, business was booming. Patients were improving and coming back for more. Intrigued, the doctor continued to prescribe the herb, but kept a check to see which conditions it helped most. He found it was effective for patients with low energy, bad coughs, pain and fatigue, and he called it 'sweet herb' because of its flavour. Gancao, its Chinese name, means sweet root. So modern research has verified an ancient story.

In Hong Kong, a herbal contraceptive may soon be developed as an inexpensive 'morning after' pill from a plant named yueh-chukene. A study at Hong Kong University showed that the wild mushroom, yun zhi, which the Chinese had been using in a tonic drink for centuries, was able to boost the T-cells, which are vital to the body's immune system. Several Chinese herbs have this ability, including *Astragalus membranaceus*, and

Ligustrum lucidum, two herbs subjected to intensive trials by research teams in China and the United States.

The root of the astragalus plant, known as huangqi, is used in about 40 per cent of all Chinese prescriptions. It is easy to obtain, and recorded in ancient books as a herb to 'build health and as a common tonic for vital energy and yin'. In modern tests it has exhibited a variety of pharmacological effects. It dilates coronary and renal arteries, has diuretic properties, and is an anti-bacterial agent. What most interests today's scientists, however, is its apparent anti-viral activity. The Chinese have long believed that a daily dose of astragalus tea prevents influenza and upper respiratory tract infections.

Western medicine has produced several impressive vaccines and antibiotics, but it seems that TCM will provide the answer to immune-system diseases like flu and cancer. Another ancient remedy for the common cold, yin qiao, is known for its ability to nip the flu bug in the bud, if sufferers take it at the first sign of symptoms.

As yet modern medicine has no modern drug to combat viral infections. China has many which were listed in the earliest book on Materia Medica, the Red Emperor's *Great Herbal*, one of the great classics of antiquity.

China's most eminent pharmacologists still refer to the Red Emperor's book, and to the celebrated *Ben Cao Gang Mu*, written by Li Shi-zhen (1518–93) because the pharmacological actions of drugs described there are helpful in current research. They have already confirmed the use of specified herbs to treat dysmenorrhoea, malaria and infections arising from insect bites and stings.

A team at the Chinese Academy of Medical Sciences has concentrated on isolating active components that have apparent anti-neo-plastic or biological response-modifier properties. An ancient prescription which in former times was used 'to purge the substantial hepatic fire' may have a role in treating myelocytic leukaemia. It is composed of eleven herbs, and is called Dan Gui Lu Hui Wan.

Researchers at Tientjin Institute of Materia Medica have isolated an active component, irisquinone, from iris pallasi seeds, commonly used to treat cancer in Chinese folk medicine. In mice, irisquinone was apparently active against tumours of the lymph gland. Another group of alkaloids extracted from a plant called *Cephalotaxus harringtonia* have been shown to inhibit tumours in mice, and to be active against two forms of leukaemia.

One of the more intriguing developments to have come out of this growing co-operation is a new willingness in the West to take note of traditional concepts. Researchers in America have pointed out that the yin-yang concept, so basic to Chinese thinking, is present in the intricate regulation and control mechanisms of the immune system. There, the suppressor (yin) and the helper (yang) T-cells are in opposition to each other, but are totally interdependent, and an imbalance of either cell population can result in disease.

Many hurdles remain before Chinese herbal medicine gains real acceptance in the West. Critics point to cases of liver toxicity in untested herbal brews, to the lack of quality control on imported substances which go into prescriptions, and to what they insist on regarding as the seemingly arcane nature of TCM theory.

Sceptics have plenty of ammunition in incidents where the wrong message has got through to the public, causing more harm than good. When ginseng was first brought to public notice, it was held up as a cure-all with near miraculous powers. Health-shop shelves were cleared of their stocks in hours, and GPs soon found their surgeries full of patients who had overdosed on ginseng when they should never have taken the herb in the first place. Ginseng is indeed a very highly prized herb, with excellent and varied properties, but like every other drug, it should only be prescribed in particular cases.

A similar incident marred the progress of trichosanthin, when early reports reached the US newspapers, suggesting it might be the cure for AIDS. Desperate victims even travelled to China to buy crude forms of the drug. Some injected it direct, and had to be given hospital treatment. In San Francisco, a gay rights group embarked on an unsupervised testing and three people subsequently died.

In ancient times, the Chinese snake gourd had been used to procure abortions, although no one knew how it worked. Research in China and Hong Kong showed that it selectively kills the trophoblast cell, which regulates activity of the placenta. The herb also targets cells in the body called macrophages (scavenger cells which clean up stray toxins).

In America, Dr Michael McGrath, director of the AIDS research laboratory in San Francisco, discovered that one of the reasons why no drug has yet been successful against AIDS is because some macrophages can be infected by the HIV virus, and the medicines so far devised killed infected T-cells, but not infected magrophages. Here at last, in a small phial given to him by Professor Yeung of Hong Kong's Chinese University, was the extract that killed the infected cells in the body's immune system, but left the healthy cells alone.

After the early press reports, and the adverse publicity which followed, trichosanthin was written off, but after four years, the drug is quietly moving through its US tests. It is probably the first Chinese drug to undergo FDA trials. It has already passed the safety trials, and if it does equally well in efficacy testing, it could be available for AIDS patients in America shortly.

If that happens, it will bring fresh hope to thousands of AIDS patients all over the world. Just as importantly, it will bring a cooperative effort between Western science and Chinese herbal knowledge into the forefront of medical advancement, with all manner of new horizons within the sight of science and humanity.

TCM defines illness as the struggle between human capability to resist disease and the pathogenic factors which cause it. Many of its herbal remedies are designed to trigger this capability. Western medicine has the technology to subject natural medicines to intensive scrutiny in the laboratory, and to reproduce them synthetically so that they can be made available to all. What better illustration of yin and yang, the two opposites which are mutually dependent and mutually supportive, could there possibly be?

CHAPTER SEVEN
Herbs and Their Uses

If you ask a typical TCM doctor why traditional Chinese medicines have such a daunting number of components, he or she will explain that a medical prescription is like a country's government: you have the Prime Minister (the active agent), the advisers (who restrain or reinforce) and the civil servants (who help the whole process to run smoothly). Or they will compare it to an orchestra, with a conductor, the various sections and the soloists. They even have a little rhyme to explain it: 'Yi jun, er chen, san zuo, si shi'; ('One ruler, two ministers, three aids and four guides'). The Chinese love to use simile and metaphor when explaining some of their customs and practices.

Pharmacology in Britain was conducted along similar lines up until relatively recently. William Hale-White's standard work, *Materia Medica*, outlined formulae which could include a *basis* (active ingredient), an *ajuvans* (to assist the active compound), a *corrigens* (to correct excess activity) and the *constituens* (the vehicle). Modern pharmacology, however, is directed towards isolating the active agent in a herb and producing a single drug.

Both systems have their drawbacks. Modern science looks askance at brews which include half a dozen ingredients of no known purpose, and critics point to recently recorded incidence of death or injury in Britain and the Continent, where people have taken herbal remedies for skin complaints, or medicine for slimming purposes. Unfortunately, though, the chemical drug industry has also had its catastrophes in recent years which far outweigh the fatalities arising from Chinese herbal concoctions.

TCM doctors constantly respond to criticism about their medicines by pointing out that these herbal prescriptions have in many cases been in daily use throughout China not just for centuries, but sometimes for thousands of years, and that in cases where people have been harmed by Chinese medicines, there have usually been other factors present which may have contributed to the outcome.

Nevertheless, it is important to sound a note of caution. The public has somehow got hold of the idea that manufactured drugs are dogged by side-effects which are inclined to be harmful, whereas 'natural' substances are not. This is a complete fallacy. Anything, taken to excess, can kill. People have turned orange and died because they had an obsessive liking for carrot juice and drank it to excess. Conversely, some people suffer from allergies which make them ill with the merest mouthful of things that can normally be eaten by the pound.

How the idea ever gained currency that all growing things were safe and benign is a complete mystery. Every summer hospital casualty wards receive a regular influx of small children who have eaten the seed cases of laburnum trees in the mistaken belief that they were peas. Digitalis, the life-saving extract which comes from the foxglove, is a poison. The Greek philosopher Socrates was condemned to death by drinking a cup of hemlock. Hamlet's uncle killed his brother by pouring a herbal brew into his ear.

All plant life must be treated with respect, and every medicine, from whatever source, should be taken with caution. Too often patients will swallow tablets prescribed for them for weeks and sometimes months on end without ever inquiring what they contain, and what possible side-effects can spring from them. It is a wise rule always to seek information on the possible side-effects of any medication, whether it comes from an orthodox or complementary practitioner.

The earliest Chinese sages referred to all medicines as poisons, not just because some of the materials they used were indeed poisonous, but basically because any substance used in treatment can 'poison' the cause of the complaint. At one time in history, doctors were reviled merely for prescribing.

Prescriptions began to be formalized after the appearance of the oldest book about herbal remedies, the famous *Ben Cao*. This is said to have been written by the ancient ruler Shen Nung, known as the Red Emperor, and sometimes called the 'Divine Husbandman' because of his knowledge of agriculture and discoveries about plants. He is acknowledged to be the father of Chinese pharmaceutics.

Shen Nung was said to have tested the effects of hundreds of plants by tasting them himself, and had been poisoned time and again. Either he possessed a remarkably robust constitution, or was a largely mythical figure, a semi-god, and his book, *The Great Herbal*, a compilation of the works of several medical authors. Legends about him say that he had a magic whisk which could alleviate the symptoms of poison, but that he did eventually succumb to poisoning and die.

Whatever its authorship, the herbal lore the book contained is said to go back 4000 years, and was the first published work to classify herbs by their pharmaceutical action. Shen Nung's list included metals and animal products, categorized in three classes: the upper class sustained life, the middle maintained the mental state, and the lower cured illness. It itemized 365 herbs for treating internal and external diseases, gynaecological disorders, eye complaints and even toothache, instructing how to prescribe, administer and process them.

This work remained the main reference source for over 1,000 years, and some of the information contained in it is still valid today. Herbs continued to be graded into the three classifications outlined in the book until the sixteenth century, when the internationally celebrated *Outline of Materia Medica* was written by Li Shi-zhen. His fifty-two volume opus listed over 2,000 medicinal plants and, 11,000 prescriptions, and classified herbs into plants, minerals and animal products, and the flora into botanical species, pre-dating similar work by Linnaeus, the Swedish botanist, by 150 years.

Since the Communist revolution in 1949, a lot of research work has been done in the medical colleges and institutes in China to identify the components in many of the most frequently used herbs, and to test their efficacy in treatment. Unfortunately, because the papers are seldom translated into foreign languages, the bulk of this data is unavailable in the West.

A very highly regarded dermatology research institution like the one at Changzheng Hospital in Tianjin has published over seventy papers and two books in recent years, and three of its research projects have won awards for advances in science and technology. They have been dispensing granular formulae instead of loose herbs for skin complaints since 1987, achieving the same results. Medical teams researching Chinese herbal treatment for skin diseases in London hospitals, and working on granular concoctions, bemoan the fact that so little clinical data is available. If this situation could be rectified, no doubt great strides could be made in mutual understanding, to the benefit of those people suffering from complaints which cannot be treated effectively by orthodox medicine.

At the Institute of Materia Medica in Beijing, they hold almost the entire Chinese 'pharmacy of nature', a collection which contains over 50,000 herbs, though only a fraction of them are in regular use. TCM doctors practising in the West will use no more than 200 or so, if that. Some which are regularly used in China are banned in Britain or prohibited through EC regulations; others have such a strong and toxic action that they can only be administered under hospital conditions where the response of the patient can be constantly monitored, and therefore cannot be used in Britain until such time as a TCM hospital is established. This will almost certainly happen eventually, given the spread of private medicine and the growing acceptance of complementary forms of treatment.

Every doctor in China, including those trained purely in Western medicine, will have spent at least one year studying herbs. Chemical drugs, even when they do not have to be imported, are often too costly to be widely used, and since medicines made from herbs can have the same effect, and are far more accessible and inexpensive, they are the logical alternative in a country where their uses and prescriptions have been tried and tested over thousands of years.

Until recent times, TCM doctors often began their long apprenticeship working on herb farms, or collecting herbs in the countryside where they lived. Herbal lore takes years of study. A doctor requires an encyclopaedic knowledge of hundreds of plants and animal products, some of which, in different species, have the same name. Even more confusingly, the same plants sometimes have a different name in different parts of the country.

Practitioners must also learn hundreds of herbal prescriptions. As an aid to memory, medical students are taught little verses, some of them thousands of years old, which help to fix the herbs and their properties, and some of the most famous prescriptions, in the mind.

In common with all other aspects of Chinese philosophy, every herb is either yin or yang, and distinguished by its property and flavour. Yang is energy, travelling upward and outward, so the action of yang herbs is directed towards the upper body and the limbs and skin. Yin herbs act internally, and have a sinking or downward motion, acting on the organs. There are four properties: cold, hot, warm or cool; and five flavours: bitter, sweet, pungent, sour, and salty. The flavour does not invariably refer to the actual taste of the herb, but to its curative nature, and as each organ is also paired with a particular taste, they are generally used to treat the organ from which the dysfunction stems.

The five flavours

Bitter herbs are used to clear heat from the body, cure coughing or vomiting, and to relieve constipation, and are used for the heart.
Sweet herbs are for the spleen, and will nourish and restore harmony, reduce pain and replenish energy.
Pungent herbs can improve the circulation and the qi, and are often used to treat relatively mild conditions. They are allied to the lungs.
Sour herbs, allied to the liver, are effective against diarrhoea, and help to stop discharge and emission.
Salty herbs also alleviate constipation and are used in the treatment of thyroid and abdominal complaints. They are connected with the kidneys.

Each herb has a 'site of action' and students are also taught that the same herb in different proportions will produce different effects. Herbs are altered by the area in which they grow. Their medicinal properties may be strengthened or weakened according to whether they are harvested in the north or the west of the country, where the soil, climate and growing conditions may be different.

The ginseng grown in Korea is different in property from the ginseng grown in America, and will be prescribed accordingly. Just as the wine produced from the Shiraz grape grown in the vineyards of France is different from the wine produced from the same type of vine in New Zealand or Chile, so the connoisseur will buy the one which he judges to be the best.

The properties of herbs are also altered in the process by which they are treated. They may be boiled, stir-fried, dried, steamed, sliced or ground, and so on, and the process can markedly change their application and influence each time, and can also transform the property of a drug from hot to cold. Coltsfoot and aster flower are much more effective at nourishing the lungs to cure a cough when stir-baked with honey, while the pain-relieving action of Corydalis tuber is greatly enhanced if it is processed with vinegar.

Medical lore passed down through millennia gives each herb its own legend and 'signature'. Doctors believe that a plant will often give outward signs of its potential for healing. Broom, for example, with its bright yellow flowers, is used in the treatment of jaundice, the characteristic symptom of which is a yellowing of the skin.

The pharmacopoeia is not restricted to plant life alone. Metals are also in regular use, though they are seldom prescribed in Britain. Cinnabar is much prized as a tranquillizer and red ochre is used to calm the liver and stop the adverse flow of qi. Dragon bones, or dinosaur fossils, often found in Shanxi, Inner Mongolia, Gansu and Hebei provinces, are also believed to induce sedation and a tranquil state of mind (though presumably not in modern-day palaeontologists). Red halloysite is used to stop chronic diarrhoea, and limonite, a type of iron ore, is used in the treatment of dysentery.

Oyster shells, dried scorpions, cuttle-fish bone and dried geckos have great value as tonics to replenish lung and kidney energy in cases of chronic asthma. Dried sea-horse is regularly used to replenish the vital function of the kidney, and is said to be effective in curing impotence.

Even the plastron (the undercarriage of a tortoise) is used to help the kidney strengthen the bones. Amber is another prized ingredient in some prescriptions. There was an old belief that when a tiger dies, its spirit enters the earth and becomes amber.

Several species of snake are used in the treatment of rheumatism and arthritis, because a snake lives in damp and wet places, but does not suffer as a result. Crushed earthworms are an effective treatment in cases of asthma. They have a similar effect to antihistamine. Dried and ground into powder, they were prescribed for patients in Tianjin First Teaching Hospital with a marked degree of success.

Toad venom, made from the dried secretion glands of two distinct species of toad, are applied externally to treat boils, ulcers and carbuncles, and swallowed for other conditions such as sore throats or tumour. Wasps' nests are applied to suppurating skin diseases, and even used as gargles. The dried body of the Chinese blistering beetle is used to remove dead tissue and accelerate the healing of wounds in cases of psoriasis, neurodermatitis, chronic ulcers and scrofula.

Items native to our own country went into the British Materia Medica not so very long ago, though we may be dismayed at the idea of taking donkey-hide gelatine, or antler horn, as Chinese patients frequently do. Westerners may have an even greater aversion to the use of powdered human afterbirth to replenish vital energy, nourish the blood and treat anaemia. They will almost certainly recoil from the idea of cooking and eating it as a meal.

In some parts of China it was apparently customary for the new parents to hold a party to celebrate the birth of a child, and to serve the placenta as an ingredient in the soup. This is a great honour for the guests, because it is thought to contain jing, the essence of life. A Western acupuncturist training in China in the 1980s was served the dish as a mark of respect, but found the taste bitter and rather strange. Fortunately, she had finished the soup before she asked for the recipe.

Today there are some twenty major classifications for herbs, some with a number of sub-classes. They are categorized according to their properties, and this is the formula followed below.

Herbs to treat exterior syndromes

ephedra
cinnamon twigs
snake-bed seed
schizonepeta
ledebouriella root
peppermint
mulberry leaf
chrysanthemum flower
pueraria root

fresh ginger
perilla leaf
wild ginger
ligusticum root
magnolia flower
xanthium fruit
centipeda herb
bupleurum root
thorowax root

arctium fruit
chaste-tree fruit
Indian chrysanthemum
 flower
cimicifuga rhizome
prepared soybean
tamarisk tops
spirodela
dichroa root

Herbs to clear internal heat

gypsum
Asian dandelion
anemarrhenia rhizome
native achyranthes root
subprostrate sophora root
blackberry lily rhizome
Chinese olive
wintercherry fruit
scandent hops
Cape jasmine fruit
berberis root
flavescent sophora root
forsythia fruit
isatis leaf
isatis root

brucea fruit
tree of heaven bark
smilax glabra rhizome
cotinus twigs
bistort rhizome
giant knotweed rhizome
gold thread
self-heal scutellarea root
coptis root
phellodendron bark
purslane
gentian root
wolfberry bark
shave grass
lophatherum

skullcap
red peony root
honeysuckle flowers
honeysuckle stem
natural indigo
dandelion herb
 viola herb
houttuynia
Paris rhizome
patrinia herb
green chiretta
oldenlandia black
 nightshade
barbat skullcap
radical lobelia

pulsatilla root
sweet wormwood
puffball
ash bark
dittany bark

reed rhizome
dogbane leaf
prunella spike
dried rehmannia root
scrophularia root

arnebia
stellaria root
swallow-wort root
imperata rhizome

Herbs to stop coughing and relieve asthma

pinellia tuber
inula flower
white mustard seed
arisaema tuber
typhonium tuber
aster root
platycodon root
trichosanthes fruit
Thunberg fritillary bulb
bitter apricot kernel
lepidium seed
perilla seed

snake gourd root
bamboo shavings
adenophora root
sargassum seaweed
laminaria
peucedanum
loquat leaf
ginko seed
coltsfoot flower
stemona root
tendrilled fritillary bulb
poppy heads

dahurian rhododendron
  leaf
lily bulb
mulberry bark
Manchurian lilac bark
boat sterculia seed
datura flower
aristolochia fruit
henbane seed
lemongrass

Purgatives

rhubarb
hemp seed
kansai root

knoxia root
genkwa flower
honey

bushcherry seed
senna leaf
aloes

Herbs to expel dampness

pubescent angelica root
tetrandra root
oriental water plantain
  rhizome
plaintain seed
lysimachia

loranthus mulberry
  mistletoe
atractylodes rhizome
oriental wormwood
cablin patchouli
round cardamom seed

agastache
amomum fruit
poria
eupatorium
katsumadai seed
tsaoko

Interior warming herbs

prepared lateral root of aconite
dried ginger
cinnamon bark
cassia bark
evodia fruit
galangal rhizome
prickly-ash peel
cloves
fennel fruit
argyi leaf
Sichuan aconite root
wild aconite root
long pepper

Herbs to regulate qi

tangerine peel
tangerine seed
immature bitter oranges
cyperus tuber
magnolia bark
macrostem onion
eagle wood
green tangerine peel
pomelo peel
bitter orange
aucklandia root

Herbs to improve appetite and digestion

germinated rice
germinated millet
hawthorn fruit
germinated barley
radish seed

Herbs to expel parasites

quisqualis fruit
areca seed
pumpkin seed
chinaberry bark
torrya seed
omphalia
carpesium fruit
carrot fruit
agrimonia bud

Herbs to stop bleeding

field thistle
sanguisorba root
hyacinth bletilla
notoginseng
cat-tail pollen
argyi leaf
small thistle
rubia root
burnet root
pagoda-tree flower
pagoda-tree flower-bud
biota tops
air-potato yam
shepherd's purse
roof stonecrop
lotus node
eclipta
patient rumex root

agrimony
Japanese thistle
imperata rhizome
boehmeria root

Herbs to promote circulation (tonify and regulate the blood)

Chuanxiong rhizome
red sage root
motherwort
corydalis tuber
curcuma root
safflower
peach kernel
achyranthes root
cyathula root

red peony root
saffron
curcuma root
turmeric
spatholobus stem
cat-tail pollen
honeylocust thorn
vaccaria seed
sappan wood

vervain
common day flower
burreed tuber
zodoary
bugle weed
pubescent holly root
frankincense
myrrh

Herbs to calm the mind and tranquillize

cinnabar
wild jujube seed
arborvitae seed
polygala root
albizia bark

albizia flower
fleece-flower stem
lucid ganoderma
valerian rhizome
mother-of-pearl

fu-shen
purple cowrie shells
oyster shell

Herbs to calm the liver

uncaria stem with hooks
gastrodia tuber

tribulus fruit
haematite

sea-ear shell

Herbs to restore consciousness

borneol

storax

grass-leaved sweet-flag rhizome

Tonic herbs

ginseng
codonopsis
astragalus root
white atractylodes
    rhizome
Chinese yam
liquorice
epimedium
eucommia bark
psoralea fruit
cistanche
Chinese angelica root

prepared rehmannia root
fleece-flower root
white peony root
glehnia root
dendrobium stem
lily bulb
wolfberry fruit
pilose asiabell root
pseudostellaria root
hedysarum root
Chinese date

Siberian solomonseal
    rhizome
malt extract
lilyturf root
asparagus root
scrophularia root
dogwood fruit
flattened milkvetch seed
glossy privet fruit

Herbs to replace lost body fluids

light wheat
schisandra fruit
black plum
lotus seeds
euryale seed
nutmeg
poppy capsule

dogwood fruit
bitter cardamom
cuttle bone
ephedra root
schisandra fruit
Cherokee rosehip
raspberry

Chinese gall
chebula fruit
pomegranate rind
lotus stamen
ginko seed

Herbs to induce perspiration

Chinese ephedra
lily-flowered magnolia
purple perilla
kudzu vine

mulberry-leafed
    chrysanthemum
ledebouriella root
perilla leaf
prepared soybean

spirodela
cassia twigs
fresh ginger
schizonepeta
pueraria root

Herbs to relieve rheumatic conditions

notopterygium root
pubescent angelica root
clematis root
large-leaf gentian root
chaenomeles fruit
siegesbeckia herb
futokadsura stem

Chinese star jasmine
acanthopanax bark
erythrina bark
vegetable sponge
common clubmoss
geranium
elder stem and leaf

glorybower leaf
Japanese dioscorea
 rhizome
paniculate swallow-wort
 root
orientvine
silkvine bark
tetrandra root

Diuretics and hydragogues

fu-ling
umbellate pore-fungus
alismatis rhizome
plantain
coix seed
Chinese wax gourd peel
areca peel
pharbitis seed
phytolacca root
croton seed
Sichuan clematis stem

Manchurian aristolochia
 stem
common knot-grass
pink
abutilon seeds
seven-lobed yam
hypoglauca yam
kansui root
dwenka flower
Peking spurge root
broom cypress fruit

lysimachia
Japanese fern spores
adsuki bean
pyrrosia leaf
calabash gourd
sweetgum fruit
corn stigma
rush pith
chamaedaphne leaf and
 flower
euphorbia root

Herbs and their channels

Herbs are also categorized according to their selective therapeutic effects on particular organs, and the meridians with which they are connected. Some may act on one channel, or several channels, and yet have no effect on others. This is called channel tropism. Certain heat-clearing herbs, for example, will act on the lung channel, and will be just as effective in treating diseases connected with the liver channel or the heart channel. Tonic herbs may be useful in strengthening the lung, yet have no effect on the spleen or the kidney.

Lung

white mustard seed	pinellia tuber	scutellaria root
ephedra	peppermint	inula flower
lily bulb	liquorice	platycodon root
glehnia root	gwenkwa flower	trichosanthes fruit
lepidium seed	hyacinth bletilla	kansui root
cinnamon twig	mulberry leaf	knoxia root
astragalus root	magnolia bark	agastache
bitter almond	Chinese yam	plantain seed
macrostem onion	chrysanthemum	ginseng
schizonepeta	scrophularia root	dried ginger
ophiopogon root	honeysuckle flower	tangerine peel
wolfberry bark	forsythia fruit	radish seed
wolfberry fruit	fritillary bulb	peach kernel
isatis leaf	gypsum	polygala root
dahurian angelica root	anemarrhenia rhizome	dangshen
perilla seed	Cape jasmine fruit	black plum

Heart

isatis leaf	coptis root	arborvitae seed
isatis root	poria	polygala root
dried rehmannia root	lateral root of aconite	grass-leaved sweet-flag rhizome
moutan bark	dried ginger	
red sage root	cinnamon bark	ginseng
motherwort	field thistle	liquorice
Manchurian aristolochia stem	corydalis tuber	Chinese angelica root
	curcuma root	ophiopogon root
fritillary bulb	safflower	lily bulb
forsythia fruit	peach kernel	light wheat
Cape jasmine fruit	wild jujube seed	lotus seed

Liver

moutan bark	white peony root	argyi leaf
red peony root	sweet wormwood	Chuanxiong rhizome
black plum	lysimachia coptis root	red sage root

dogwood fruit
schizonepeta
cuttle bone
fleece-flower root
 loranthus mulberry
    mistletoe
dried rehmannia root
peppermint
mulberry leaf
chrysanthemum
rhubarb
bupleurum root
gentian root

plantain seed
oriental wormwood
cinnamon bark
evodia fruit
motherwort
corydalis tuber
cyperus tuber
germinated barley
field thistle
sanguisorba root
hyacinth bletilla
notoginseng
cat-tail pollen

curcuma root
safflower
peach kernel
achyranthes and cyathula
    root
wild jujube seed
uncaria stem with hooks
gastrodia tuber
epimedium
eucommia bark
Chinese angelica root
wolfberry fruit

Spleen

pinellia tuber
radish seed
ledebouriella root
aucklandia root
atractylodes rhizome
amomum fruit
poria
pueraria root
rhubarb
bushcherry seed
inula flower
agastache

oriental wormwood
lateral root of aconite
quisqualis fruit
cinnamon bark
evodia fruit
tangerine peel
immature bitter orange
hawthorn fruit
psoralea fruit
germinated barley
cordyalis tuber
curcuma root

ginseng
dangshen
astragalus root
white atractylodes
    rhizome
Chinese yam
black plum
liquorice
Chinese angelica root
white peony root
lotus seed
bitter cardamom

Kidney

moutan bark
kansui root
knoxia root
desert cistanche
pubescent angelica root
loranthus mulberry
    mistletoe

gwenka flower
sweet wormwood
oriental water plantain
    rhizome
plantain seed
anemarrhenia rhizome
tetrandra root

cinnamon bark
argyi leaf
achyranthes and cyathula
    root
bitter cardamom
arborvitae seed
Chinese yam

lysimachia
notopterygium root
dried rehmannia root
wolfberry bark
wolfberry fruit
scrophularia root

phellodendron bark
poria
umbellate pore fungus
lateral root of aconite
eucommia bark
psoralea fruit

dendrobium stem
epimedium
fleece-flower root
lotus seed
dogwood fruit
cuttle bone

Bladder

ephedra
pubescent angelica root
ledebouriella root
notopterygium root
lepidium seed

tetrandra root
umbellate pore-fungus
oriental water plantain rhizome

Manchurian aristolochia stem
lysimachia
motherwort

Stomach

honeysuckle flower
pinellia tuber
hemp seed
mirabilite
dahurian angelica root
atractylodes rhizome
isatis leaf
scrophularia root
gypsum
white atractylodes rhizome
macrostem onion
hawthorn fruit
anemarrhenia rhizome

Cape jasmine fruit
Scutellaria root
coptis root
inula flower
trichanthes fruit
agastache
dried ginger
amomum fruit
oriental wormwood
evodia fruit
ophiopogon root
immature bitter orange
aucklandia root
magnolia bark

germinated barley
radish seed
quisqualis fruit
areca seed
pumpkin seed
glehnia root
sanguisorba root
hyacinth bletilla
notoginseng
grass-leaved sweet-flag rhizome
liquorice
dendrobium stem
cuttle bone

Gallbladder

bupleurum root
scutellaria root
gentian root

forsythia fruit
sweet wormwood
lysimachia

oriental wormwood
aucklandia root
Chuanxiong rhizome

San jiao
Cape jasmine fruit   cyperus tuber

Pericardium
Chuanxiong rhizome   red sage root   uncaria stem with hooks
cat-tail pollen

Large intestine
inula flower   perilla seed   areca seed
hemp seed   rhubarb   pumpkin seed
scutellaria root   mirabilite   genkwa flower
coptis root   bushcherry seed   immature bitter orange
phellodendron bark   aucklandia root   sanguisorba root
honeysuckle flower   kansui root   peach kernel
pulsatilla root   knoxia root   arborvitae seed
triocanthes fruit   magnolia bark   desert cistanche
bitter almond kernel   macrostem onion   black plum

Small intestine
bushcherry seed   Manchurian aristolochia stem

CHAPTER EIGHT
Eating for Health the Chinese Way

'Food is a medicine and medicine is food', runs a well-known Chinese proverb. Not, perhaps, one which people who have taken herbal medicines in their raw form will feel too enthusiastic about, but perfectly true, nevertheless.

Modern-day nutritionists are constantly telling us that a balanced diet is the best way to keep healthy. In the *Nei Jing*, three centuries before the birth of Christ, the Yellow Emperor advised a daily intake of cereal grains, meats, fruits and vegetables. Confucius also handed out dietary advice which would meet with the full approval of twentieth-century nutritionists.

Primitive people's understanding of the medical properties of the food they ate evolved through the centuries, as they gradually observed that when certain ingredients were in the cooking pot, there was a noticeable effect on their health and well-being. Perhaps their headache eased after eating, or they began to vomit. Maybe their fever abated, their joint pain eased, or they got diarrhoea.

Once people began to suspect an association between such physical effects and the particular ingredient or ingredients responsible, they started to isolate them to treat specific ailments, but they continued to include them in food, as a way of sustaining and maintaining good health, and this still continues today.

Around 1700 BC, in the Shong Dynasty, a legendary cook came to work in the Emperor's kitchens. His name was I-Yin, and he learned exactly what herbs were best included in court dishes to produce beneficial medicinal effects. The herb soups which continue to feature so widely in the Chinese diet were devised by I-Yin. He was said to be the first to dispense medicinal decoctions and he could be called the first dietician. Some histories claim he was actually the Prime Minister, but the story of Chinese medicine and the hallowed figures who contributed to its development is often vague on these points.

In the fourteenth century, Hu Si-hui, a Mongolian who had been chef of the imperial household of the Yuan Dynasty, compiled a textbook based on his experience in the royal kitchens and his knowledge of herbal medicines, entitled *Principles of Correct Diet*, which he presented to the Emperor. In a food-and-health-conscious country, there could be no better gift.

Ideally, we should eat only to relieve hunger, and drink to ease thirst, but no nation enjoys eating a well-cooked and skilfully prepared meal more than the Chinese. It is their custom to regale guests with banquets which literally turn the table into a groaning board. Dish after dish will arrive at the table, where the host personally heaps food on to the plates of the guests; delicacies served first while the appetite is still sharp, and rice and soup to round off the meal.

All meals, sumptuous or plain, will be balanced by both 'fan' and 'ts'ai' dishes. Fan includes rice, cereals or starchy dishes, ts'ai originally meant vegetables, but has come to designate the accompanying meat or fish dishes.

At home, the Chinese often treat a minor ailment with a specially prepared meal, or by including a particular ingredient in a dish. When her family return from work shivering in the bitter winds of a Beijing winter, a housewife will pour them a warming cup of spring onion tea, to chase the chill out of their bones and prevent the onset of a cold. If someone is suffering from stomach discomfort or nausea, they will drink tea made from ginger, which is a warming herb and very effective against both these complaints. Ginger is also a detoxicant. Anyone who suspects their stomach pains may be the onset of food poisoning, could make themselves a tea with several ounces of fresh ginger (the more the better) and it will help to alleviate the symptoms. Liquorice can help to stop colic pains; it is often prescribed, with peony root, for tummy ache in children.

A victim of Parkinson's disease might be served the steamed feet of a black-legged chicken, which is regarded as a great blood-purifier. Even if we felt inclined to try the dish in the West, it would be difficult to find the ingredients in our factory-farmed, homogenized society, but learning the Chinese philosophy of food is a worthwhile exercise and there are many homespun folk medicine recipes which are made from foodstuffs found in any kitchen, and are well worth trying.

Yin and yang foods

Balance and harmony are paramount in preparing a meal or planning a diet. In Chinese terms, almost every foodstuff is either yin, which is cool or cold in property, or yang, which is warm or hot. When a Chinese doctor advises a patient to avoid hot or cold foods, he doesn't mean the temperature at which they are served, but the actual classification of the ingredients themselves. This is another of those ostensibly strange oriental theories which make immediate sense when put into Western terms: as a general rule, the greater the calorific value of a food item, the 'hotter' it is likely to be considered in the Chinese dietary code. Thus fatty flesh, alcohol and peanuts are all hot foods. Fruits, seaweeds and green vegetables are cold.

Raw foods are rarely eaten in China. Even in summer, salad vegetables are likely to be cooked very briefly – a sensible precaution in a country with extremes of climate, where summer can be intensely hot and humid, and where fresh, clean water is not always on tap. Modern Chinese think that the Western diet, with its emphasis on long-cooked, rich foods, simply invites 'hot' diseases like flu.

It is common practice in the UK to serve cucumber raw in salads. In most parts of China, it is usually cooked. This is because it is categorized as cold in property, and the body will have to use up its own energy to warm it. If you think about this, it makes sound practical sense in both Eastern and Western terms. A cucumber contains very few calories, and is inclined to be rather indigestible, so the gastric system has to work extra hard to metabolize it.

The Chinese see no point in eating a food which provides one calorie of energy, if it takes two calories of energy to process it. Therefore, they steam or stir-fry cucumber, thereby ensuring that the effort needed to digest it is provided by the cooking process, rather than the body. Older people will make sure that their diet does not include 'cold' meals, since they will deplete their internal energy by eating them. Uniquely Chinese dishes like bird's nest soup, shark's fin and ginseng are considered to be strengthening dishes and so is carrot, the seeds of which are commonly used to treat cases of dysentery.

Foodstuffs which grow in spring and summer are generally cooling in quality, and the Chinese, as part of a philosophy based on nature and the natural laws, believe that ideally diet should always be planned around fresh produce in season. Salads, cucumbers and leafy vegetables are summer foods. Most root vegetables, red meat, and ginger, so integral to Chinese cuisine, are warm foods for autumn and winter dishes.

Cooking methods will alter the yin or yang nature of produce. Water is always considered to have a cooling influence, even when it is used for boiling or steaming. Cooking by fire – roasting, grilling or baking – will make food hot. A hen's egg, which is warm in property, will become cool if it is boiled. A duck's egg, on the other hand, which is designated a cool food because a duck spends much of its time in water, will become warm if it is fried.

Fish is self-evidently cold, since its natural environment is water, and therefore it is invariably cooked with ginger, to warm up the dish and give it balance. Shellfish, however, which live entirely in water, are categorized as hot, because of their shells, and certain types of shellfish, which live in shallow water, are considered to have toxic qualities, or what the Chinese call poison heat. Anyone suffering from boils, or recovering from surgery, will be told to avoid crab and prawns for this reason. The poison heat could set up an infection in stitches. Lobster, however, which comes from deeper waters, is not considered a danger in this way.

Even noodles belong to opposite categories, according to whether they are made from rice or wheat. Rice grows in water, and products made from it are cool. Wheat, which ripens in the sun, is hot. So in addition to ensuring that a meal has the right balance of yin and yang, a good cook will also take care that the 'climate' of the meal is balanced.

As with herbs, the Chinese take note of the 'signature' of a food item. Walnuts nourish the brain, they believe, because of the resemblance the nut has to the brain. A pig's tail strengthens the spine in growing children.

Chinese food is one of the world's major cuisines, yet it was created through the ages in a famine-ravaged land, and inspired by the logistics of starvation. Even when times were better, there was a shortage of pastureland and very rarely any surplus grain to spare for animal fodder. Beef was therefore a rarity and dairy products virtually unknown.

Pork became the most familiar meat because pigs were very cheap to keep and to feed. They can forage in woodland on nuts and acorns and were also fed the water in which rice was washed. Chickens and ducks were equally economical to rear, and duck and chicken meat remains a regular ingredient in many folk medicines.

It was through the survival techniques learned in the lean years that Chinese cuisine developed its unique character. Until relatively recently, food vendors peeled oranges and sold the skins separately as flavouring for dishes or for preserving. Cooks made the smallest portion of meat feed an entire family by cutting it into slivers. Bean sprouts, beancurd and pulses supplied much of the necessary protein. The wok is the most efficient cooking utensil ever devised for the dispersal of heat; little fuel is required for it, it needs only small amounts of cooking oil, and the stir-frying technique which epitomizes Chinese cooking ensures that vegetables retain all their vitamins and flavour and stay crisp and appetizing.

Herb soups

One of the main health tonics that Chinese housewives will always have on hand are herb soups, which they use to tonify the body whenever anyone is ill or out of sorts, or convalescing. The Chinese word 'tang' is the collective term for soup, and herbal factories in China supply specially prepared herbal tang to hospitals and clinics all over the country. In Britain, these ready-made formulas are sold in Chinese supermarkets, and the list includes about fifty different varieties.

Since it is an integral part of their culture, the Chinese know precisely which tang will best help their recovery. In Zhang Zhong-jing's celebrated classic on the treatment of febrile diseases, he recommended a soup of Chinese angelica root, fresh ginger and mutton, and another made with lily bulb and the yolk of egg, which are still known today, and are served in the medicated diet dining halls which are sometimes attached to hospitals. One hospital in Chengdu, in Sichuan province, has a dining hall with ninety-six medicated diet recipes, devised for patients suffering from conditions such as diabetes, obesity and heart problems.

Those who are convalescing at home will make their own tonic broths, choosing the ingredients according to their known therapeutic qualities. Lily bulb is said to nourish the lungs, clear away fire in the heart and have a calming effect on the mind. Chinese angelica is a blood tonic, frequently used to help women with period problems.

Everyone in China automatically eats this way, and broths are quite simple to prepare. For example, a couple of free-range, corn-fed chicken breasts, slowly simmered in a bain-marie until the meat has broken down, will ensure that the nourishment from the chicken goes into the water. Someone with no appetite, or unable to take solids, will get all the goodness of the chicken merely by drinking the broth.

A tonic gruel made with pork kidney, polished rice, scallions, fresh ginger and five-spice powder, eaten each morning for breakfast is said to be helpful for old people suffering from loss of hearing, lassitude and weakness in the legs. In the elderly, declining powers are regarded as a kidney deficiency.

Tea

Many scholars believe that tea was originally used as a medicine. Throughout modern China, from the simplest homes to the plushest of the new Western-style hotels, a large thermos flask is replenished with tea morning and evening. Everyone sips tea all day long, in cups with lids to hold the heat in. Cold water is rarely drunk, another sensible health precaution in overcrowded cities where many homes still do not have running water. Some varieties of tea have strange names like 'Old Man's Eyebrows' and there are shops devoted entirely to selling tea, from local specialities to luxury brands from the far corners of the country. This possibly accounts for the popularity of tea-houses in China, those happy havens were men were entertained by poetry, story-telling and courtesans who went by the name of sing-song girls.

Tea continues to be drunk for its health-giving properties. Some teas will be recommended as aids to digestion, some for weight loss, others as tonics and general pick-me-ups. They are certainly expected to have more benefits for the drinker than the merely restorative qualities of a British cuppa.

Proscribed foods

Traditional doctors working in the West are treating patients in a completely different culture, where diet is still based on large quantities of meat and dairy products, plus refined and processed foodstuffs, and the careful TCM doctor makes sure that prescriptions are amended accordingly. This is because the food we eat can affect the action of the herbs in medicines, and dietary advice should always be given to ensure that the medicine is not impeded or affected by the patient's own eating habits.

People suffering from eczema, which is a blood heat condition, will be advised not to eat anything which is cooked by direct fire. They will be asked to limit themselves to dishes which can be steamed, boiled and – just occasionally – stir-fried, instead of roasted, grilled, or baked foods.

No one with a temperature should eat spicy food, because that will simply make the situation worse. People who lack energy and constantly feel tired, should avoid foods that burn up energy even more quickly – garlic, carrots, even mustard seeds are considered by the Chinese to belong to this category. Those whose illness is diagnosed as the result of dampness will be advised not to eat cheese, or to take too much sugar or salt. Sugar or salt left in a bowl will quickly turn damp and sticky, and Chinese physicians contend that they will do precisely the same thing in the human body.

Hot and cold foods

Most dietary guidelines are derived from nature. The way an animal lives or a plant grows has a major influence on the way it is categorized. Lamb is a hot food, which gives a lot of yang energy, and would never be eaten in the summer. Sheep thrive in a cold climate, because they have a woolly fleece to protect them, and in Beijing, on the first day of autumn, people dine on lamb dishes, to build up their reserves of fat before the winter sets in and the biting cold sweeps in from the Mongolian steppes. Wild game is the hottest food of all, and is eaten in vast amounts in winter. Wild boar, venison, pheasant and rabbit all feature regularly on the menus of health-conscious families in China when the winter sets in. Chicken is a neutral food, and so are most of the grains which it eats. Pork is cool in nature: the meat is paler in colour and the pig rather enjoys a wallow in mud.

Diet and women's health

Diet is considered to be an especially vital factor in the well-being of women (climate and stress are considered to be the other main culprits in gynaecological problems). The menstrual cycle involves a monthly depletion of energy through blood loss, and the food eaten before and during a period should compensate for that. Unless a woman ensures that she is well nourished, her zhong qi – the pool of energy held in the centre of the body between the stomach and the spleen – will be deficient, and she will be unable to replenish her reserves.

Fibroids, for example, are diagnosed as cold in the uterus, exacerbated by poor diet. A TCM practitioner would advise any vegetarian woman patient to avoid salads and raws foods, and to stick to eating cooked meals, preferably using vegetables and pulses that are in the warm or neutral category. Cabbage is regarded as a particularly cold food, and should certainly be avoided in such cases.

Diet in pregnancy

As is well known, diet is extremely important in pregnancy, but it has a special relevance for the Chinese with their philosophical reverence for inheritance and ancestry. The food an expectant mother eats will, they say, directly affect the 'before heaven energy' which she bequeaths to the foetus in the womb. This is a sacred gift, and finite in quantity. The amount she provides the infant with must last the child throughout its life. Therefore, she will ensure that her diet includes plenty of nutritious fish and neutral items, and will avoid any extreme tastes, such as very hot or very cold foods, and spicy dishes which can cause heat and, according to TCM doctors, could result in the baby developing skin problems after birth. As the foetus develops in the womb, the diet changes to take account of alterations in the mother's body.

The first three months of pregnancy involve eating warming foods, and tonic dishes such as pork, steamed rice and tan-kuei (an angelica herbal tonic), but in three to six months cool foods will be introduced to counter the hot conditions which prevail in the uterus during the final months before the birth, and expectant mothers will cut down on the tonic foods to reduce the danger of a large baby and a difficult birth. Chilli and alcohol are avoided as it is believed they can bring on miscarriage.

One of the great standbys of pregnancy and post-natal care is ginger. A cupful of warm tea, made by slicing or grating a 5-cm/2-in piece of fresh ginger into freshly boiled water, and leaving it to stand until the juices have been thoroughly absorbed into the water, is a safe and reliable antidote to morning sickness.

China has a few old wives' tales, just like the rest of the world. In some parts of the country, expectant mothers will avoid lamb or mutton dishes, not because they are considered hot dishes, but because their name is very similar to the word for epilepsy.

After a baby is born, a woman's diet and routine becomes crucially important. A new mother will avoid washing her hair for the first month after the birth. It is universally agreed that heat loss is always greatest through the head, but the Chinese have another reason for protecting the top of the head. The acupoint there is one of the most important on the body. The liver is the principal organ involved in childbirth and pregnancy, and the liver meridian and the governor vessel channel meet at a point in the top of the head. Labour is considered to bring on a cold imbalance, so when the energy pool is low after birth, a woman will not do anything that might let further cold invade her body. She will not even take a bath, but will simply wipe herself with a warm cloth.

Another custom involves eating as many eggs as possible in the first month following the birth. A Western writer living in the Beijing area during the early 1920s recorded that women able to afford it would eat four to six eggs a day. Eggs contain protein, and the new mother will ensure that she has other things in her diet so that this high intake of eggs does not cause constipation.

Rebuilding strength after the cold imbalance brought on by labour is considered of the utmost importance. It is called 'doing the month', and the practice still continues in many parts of China. In the early weeks a woman will remain inside her home and rest in bed as much as possible. She will tonify her system with ginger stews. These are made with pounds of ginger, peeled and crushed and then covered with a special sweet vinegar and simmered for hours until the liquid has reduced and the goodness of the ingredients mingled into a sweet-tasting and delicious gravy. This is then kept as the stock, which will be used to stew chicken, duck or perhaps a little pork, and very often pigs' feet, as a main meal each day. A special chicken soup includes ginger, peanuts, dried jujubes and rice wine.

Any new mother whose milk supply is inadequate will make a soup using a whole carp, or St Peter's fish if carp is not available. Into the pot will go also a box of silken tofu, with ginger and salt to taste. After it is brought to the boil and simmered for an hour, the soup resembles milk, and is said to be very effective in improving lactation.

Ginger warms the spleen and the stomach, and is also an excellent detoxicant against any germs likely to cause food poisoning, which is one of the reasons why it is always used as an ingredient in fish dishes. Ginger and tangerine peel counterbalance each other, and are included in several everyday recipes, as well as being regular ingredients in any number of effective prescriptions. Tangerine peel dries dampness in the spleen and is used to alleviate catarrh or a tendency to diarrhoea.

In China, all children are considered to have a weak spleen and an 'excessive' liver, because their bodies are still developing. This is the cause of a lot of colic and digestive problems. One homespun antidote to this is the residue of rice which sticks to the bottom of the pan when it has caught slightly during the cooking process. A Chinese mother will pour water into the pan to boil this, and make it into a tea for her baby. It is believed to soothe the stomach and aid digestion. Sesame seeds are good to nourish the blood, and a tablespoonful sprinkled over food is an easy tonic for old and young alike.

Cystitis

Doctors working in the West are aware of British squeamishness and are reluctant to advise simple remedies which they would have no hesitation in recommending to patients at home. One Chinese doctor, who runs a busy London practice as well as contributing to the research work into herbal medicines at the Royal Free Hospital, is usually at pains to stress the modern scientific credentials of Chinese medicine. However, when a patient came to him desperate to find a cure for the recurrent cystitis that was ruining her sex life, he overcame inbuilt caution about making TCM sound arcane and mystical, and gave her the advice a country practitioner in China would give his patients: find a butcher who will sell a sheep's bladder, fill it with a handful of peppercorns, boil for one hour, then drink the juice.

She managed to find the ingredients, and the remedy did the trick. However, it should be borne in mind that this remedy is strictly for women suffering from recurrent cystitis, commonly called 'honeymoon cystitis'. It is important that anyone suffering from acute cystitis, arising from an infection, immediately seeks treatment from a GP.

Acute cystitis may be eased by drinking a tea made from the common plantain herb which grows so profusely in grass and on lawns. In China, half a pound of plantain, either the whole grass or the seed, is washed, cleaned and boiled for about fifteen minutes and the tea drunk regularly until the trouble clears.

Folk medicine recipes

External

Abscess: Apply a lotion of rhubarb and peony flowers ground down, mixed together with sesame oil.
Mastitis: Applications of powdered, dry rhubarb root mixed with olive oil will ease discomfort and hasten healing.
Minor burns: Shake on a few drops of soy sauce.
Mosquito bites: Smear on palm oil.
Pimples and spots: Cleanse skin with a slice of fresh watermelon. Rheumatoid arthritis: Powdered rhubarb root mixed with sesame oil is used as an ointment.

Internal

Bed-wetting: Chicken gizzard is used in southern China as a remedy for children who wet their bed. You powder and cook it first, then sprinkle it over a lunch or dinner dish, so that they are hardly aware of what they are eating. It is said to work in many instances, and is certainly a good deal less traumatic for a little one than a mattress cover which sounds an alarm bell. In Northern China, chicken gizzard is also used to treat children with worms. It can be bought in some Chinese herb shops.
Constipation in the elderly: Pears stewed in honey.

Teas

Tension headaches: Take the white parts of three or four spring onions, and boil in a mugful of water. Drink the juice.

Tonsillitis: A generous handful of honeysuckle flowers, boiled in a mugful of water and drunk regularly, should ease discomfort. Take the pulp of two fresh pomegranates, soak in boiling water for thirty minutes, then wrap in a piece of antiseptic gauze and wring out the juice. It can be used several times a day as a gargle. Salt water is also recommended as a gargle. Spicy foods should be avoided.

CHAPTER NINE
Qi Gong

In a basement gym in South Kensington, a class of nine students begins the breathing exercises which are the preliminary feature of qi gong. Eight men and one woman stand motionless, listening to the soft voice of their teacher intoning instructions, while gentle music flows almost imperceptibly through the sound system to provide a tranquil background for their concentration. It looks a very tame affair; but not for long.

Slowly, from somewhere in the hall, a noise begins. It starts as a low hum, and then grows into a persistent animal sound, pitched between a moan and a whine. Unearthly, and apparently untraceable, it is difficult to pinpoint which of the people there is making it, if indeed it has any human provenance at all. No one gives any sign of having heard, no one seems to be responsible for it.

But then the sound increases by several decibels, deepening to a growl and then a groan, and suddenly a young man in his twenties drops on all-fours and begins to imitate the actions of a tiger. His qi (the invisible energy within him) has taken over. In a trance-like state, his movements are no longer his own.

Gradually, the others in the room become possessed in a similar way. One mimics the delicate steps of a deer, pressing his hands against the sides of his temples as if they are antlers. The woman begins to flutter her arms as if they are the wings of a bird. Another man drops to the floor and begins a frantic drumming motion, before switching to slapping his own head with a force which must surely inflict considerable pain.

There is something at once alarming and amusing about watching this particular form of qi gong for the first time. It looks like something children might play at kindergarten, or a study in one of the more extreme forms of method acting. To the participants, however, this is serious work. According to their teacher, the class had reached the stage where their qi could take over their bodies and dictate their movements.

The particular form of qi gong they are following is an offshoot of a system devised by the famous physician Hua Tuo, who spent many hours observing the way animals moved in the wild, and believed that man could benefit from copying them. He taught his pupils, 'When one is physically active, the energy that one takes in with food becomes available for use, the bodily fluids can circulate without hindrance, and sickness cannot take hold – just like the hinge of a door which always turns but never rusts. The ancient immortals devised certain exercises, bending and stretching, imitating the stance of the climbing bear, or the owl swivelling its head, as well as rotating the pelvis and flexing all the other joints.'

Hua was said to be nearly 100 when he met his end. One of his two pupils (both of whom also became famous doctors) diligently practised the exercises his master taught him and was reported to have lived to over ninety, retaining perfect teeth, eyesight and hearing.

The system the class is following also pairs the animals with five emotions. When they begin, under the force of the qi, to move like either the tiger, the deer, the monkey, the bear or the bird, it is not merely the animal they are imitating. They are also acting out the real emotions that they feel within. Their teacher explained: 'One of my students may come here believing that he is sad about something, whereas in actual fact he is angry. When his qi takes over, he cannot lie, even to himself. The animal which reflects his true feelings will come through.'

In Britain, such displays seem hardly credible. In China, qi gong is one of the mainstays of everyday life. In early morning, in city parks and squares, even in the biting cold of winter, men and women of all ages stand practising their own form of qi gong, often the graceful, languid movements of tai qi, which is one of its derivatives.

Fundamentally, qi gong is a method of meditational exercise aimed at cultivating physical and spiritual perfection. There are dozens – some say hundreds – of different forms, many still being evolved by present-day qi gong masters; but they all spring from the same ancient root, and all are based on the meridians which interconnect the internal organs and viscera with the exterior of the body, through which the qi flows.

The meditational forms, which require stillness, belong to the category of qi gong called nei dan, and involve standing motionless, sitting or lying. The active forms, wei dan, involve exercises basically intended to cultivate physical fitness and strength, but always with a spiritual element. Ideally, all forms are best practised out of doors, preferably in a tranquil and beautiful setting, so that one can be inspired by nature, which is always in a transitional state, and yet constant.

One of its main precepts concerns finding the centre of the body, to attain perfect balance as a prerequisite to health. Students will be taught to visualize the soles of their feet reaching hundreds of yards deep down into the earth, or a rod passing down their spine via the centre of their head and penetrating deep into the ground. Once they achieve that, no one will be able to knock them off balance. It proves that the qi is perfectly centred, neither too weak in one part of the body nor too strong in another.

Some of those going through the movements in the dawn light will be moving like the clouds, constantly changing but without the appearance of change. Others will stand close to a tree, whose topmost branches are in the sky and whose roots reach down into the centre of the earth.

It is fascinating to watch this daily ritual in the parks and squares, each person absorbed in their own concentration, moving with a balletic grace and fluidity of movement. According to the *Nei Jing*, the spiritual beings who inhabited the planet in ancient times and who lived such long and peaceful lives were like trees: 'They stood between heaven and earth, connecting the universe. They inhaled the vital essence of life. They remained unmoving in their spirit. Their muscles and flesh were as one. This is the Tao, the Way you are looking for.'

The Tao, the Way of nature, is at the heart of Chinese philosophy. (It is discussed further in the Appendix.) Those who live according to its rules will achieve longevity, health and serenity. There is a saying that if a person lives by the Tao, and dies at 120, he dies young. What is meant by this is that peace of mind and good health are a natural consequence of living simply and keeping fit by practising physical and spiritual exercises. Someone who leads a serene and healthy life is very likely to live to a great age. Age is therefore venerated and respected because it is an indication of living according to the Tao.

No people are more health-conscious than the Chinese, born into a culture which emphasizes that personal responsibility for one's own well-being is paramount. This involves taking care of the three Tan T'ien, the three cavities of the body in which the Three Treasures are stored and cultivated. The essence is stored in the lower abdomen, the emotions and energy reside in the centre of the abdomen, and mental and spiritual dimensions are cultivated in the head.

The Three Treasures are jing (essence), qi (energy) and shen (spirit). People are taught from childhood that their genetic jing energy must be protected and nurtured. If they overtax themselves with work, or indulge in too much drink or sex, they will not only deplete this inherited reserve of health and strength, but pass on that weakness to the next generation.

Their second pool of energy is the everyday zest and stamina which can flag from time to time when life becomes stressful or demanding. This can be topped up when it becomes depleted; but if it is well maintained at all times, then this is much less likely to happen.

The spirit has a more physical aspect than the Western concept. It is nourished by qi, even though it is on a higher level. During the waking hours, the spirit resides in the head. Its true home, however, is the heart, into which it returns at night.

All qi gong exercises are based on the Chinese concept of physiology. Anyone learning the system must first understand the way this works. Qi circulates around the meridians, the invisible lines which connect the outer surface of the body to the internal organs. Acupuncture works by needling these lines at specific points to balance the energy of the organs and the viscera, but those who reach true proficiency in qi gong will be able to achieve precisely the same effect by the power of the mind.

Certain of these points are central to qi gong practice. These are the navel, the crown, the brow, the tongue, the heart, the palms of the hand, the kidney, the perineum and the sole of the foot.

There are three other divisions of the torso, known as the Three Chou, which divide into the area below the navel, from the navel to the base of the rib-cage, and from the diaphragm to the neck. Each governs the internal organs of its own area, and operates at a different temperature. The right balance between them must always be maintained.

Chinese children grow up absorbing this knowledge from the cradle. Every child is taught that falling ill can often be caused by self-neglect; good health will result from living sensibly and taking proper care of both body and mind. For that reason, at least 60 million people in mainland China start each day with a form of exercise which does not aim to burn off energy, but rather to accrue, store and reinforce it.

Qi gong is the forefunner of TCM, since qi, the subtle breath, or life energy, is at the heart of everything. In the human body there are two forms of qi, the yin qi which refers to vitality, and the yang qi which is resistance to disease. Gong, loosely translated, means achievement, implying that by long practice, the qi can be cultivated and harmonized to maintain health, serenity and vigour, and in some cases, bestow superhuman qualities on the true master.

The system is thought to have been pre-eminent in the days of the alchemists, those early pseudo-scientists who searched for the elixir of eternal life, and deduced that the best way to find it would be to harness and control the energy that created and sustained all existence. Under their influence, the purity of Taoism as a philosophy became imbued with all manner of superstitious practices, and overlaid with religious ones.

The spiritual perfection and mental tranquillity which came with meditation were intended to free the body from earthly desires, and, rather like the Buddhist idea of Nirvana, to enable it to escape from the prison of the flesh to a state where it could emulate the powers of the spiritual beings and travel the universe at will. This was the Way, the life of purity, one of whose natural consequences was a long and blissful existence. The Taoist alchemists, however, saw things rather differently. They searched for a potion which would give them life everlasting.

One of these men, Chang Tao-Ling, who wrote a book of charms, was known as the Taoist Pope. He declared that 'feeding the soul so that it does not die is the acquisition of the celestial breath with the female terrestrial breath. In using them, no exertion is to be made.' Legend relates that he was given the elixir of life supernaturally by Lao Tzu, and survived until the age of 123, whereupon he swallowed the elixir and ascended into the heavens to dwell with the immortals.

Another of the Taoist alchemists, Chuang Tzu (Tzu is an honorary title, meaning 'Master') declared: 'Blowing and gasping, sighing and breathing, expelling old breath and taking in the new. Passing time like the dormant bear, stretching and bending the neck like a bird, all these show the desire for longevity. This is done by the doctors who inhale and the men who nourish their bodies.'

Pao Po Tzu advised: 'Breathe, through the nose, hold the breath and mentally count the heartbeats. Count to 120 then exhale through the mouth. You should not hear the sound. Inhale generously, exhale sparingly. Suspend a wild goose feather in front of the nose and the mouth. The feather should not stir.

'With long practice, the breath may be held for 1,000 beats. At that stage, an old man will be transformed into a young man; each day adding to the transformation.' Having the power and potency of youth even into old age was obviously a highly desirable acquisition.

In the centuries since, qi gong has been refined into the martial arts and meditational exercises, as well as a system for promoting physical strength and well-being. But its first recorded appearance is in the *Nei Jing*, where the Yellow Emperor asks his divine teacher: 'I have heard that in ancient times the people lived to be over 100 years, and yet they did not become decrepit in their activities. Nowadays people reach only half that age and yet become decrepit and failing. Is it because the world changes from generation to generation? Or is mankind becoming negligent of the laws of nature?'

The teacher replied that they lived natural lives and were content with little. 'They exercised restraint of their will and reduced their desires, their hearts were at peace and without fear. Their bodies toiled and yet did not become weary.'

The book advises: 'Exhale and inhale the essence qi, concentrate the spirit to keep a sound mind, then the muscles and the flesh unite as one.'

In 1973, archaeologists excavating a 2,100-year-old tomb from the Western Han Dynasty, near the village of Mawangdui in Hunan province, discovered a series of medical textbooks printed on silk, which contained references to drawing nutrition from the air instead of food.

Many of the earliest physicians and monks practised and developed their own forms of qi gong. One revered teacher Da Mo, an Indian prince who went to China to preach Buddhism, was said to have lived nine years as a hermit in a monastery, while he worked out a system to improve the health of the weak and sickly monks he found there. When he emerged, he taught them how to use the qi to wash out their own bone marrow to enliven the blood cells and nourish the brain. This way their bodies would become invincible and they would also achieve enlightenment. This system became integrated into the martial arts, and the Shaolin Temple, in Hunan province, remains famous for Da Mo's discoveries even to this day.

Another famous form was created by a marshal, Yeuh Fei, in order to maintain the strength and stamina of his soldiers. The set of exercises he developed is known as the Eight Pieces of Brocade.

Qi gong was suppressed in China for ten years during the Cultural Revolution, possibly because of its close connection with warfare. It has always been used by fighting men to build up their strength, and there are stories and legends about experts who could engage in battle merely by standing motionless and projecting their qi toward their enemy.

Like most of the country's ancient traditions, qi gong refused to die out. It always had a secret, spiritual aspect which was passed down the generations from father to son, or from a master to a favoured pupil. These secrets were never written down, in case they fell into the wrong hands. At the end of the 1970s it came back into favour, and was recognized as part of the cultural heritage and one of the country's 'national treasures'. Various scientific organizations have since been set up to research and investigate qi gong. Research carried out in a Beijing hospital showed that qi gong exercise made the heartbeat slow down and strengthened its action. The capillaries dilated, increasing blood circulation, haemoglobin levels rose, the protein in red cells was significantly increased, resulting in greater absorption of oxygen, and the blood pressure was lowered.

Today in China, qi gong has reached cult status. More books are written and sold on the subject than any other. People wait for months to be taught by the best masters, hoping to find anything from inner tranquillity to a cure for a back pain. Present-day Grand Masters who have reached the higher realms of the art are said to be able to transmit their qi to bring water to the boil merely by holding a hand in front of the glass, or to throw a cup in the air and suspend it there for minutes by the force of the qi that emanates from their outstretched palm. All this may sound like the Chinese equivalent of the Indian rope trick, but many rational, sceptical and otherwise reliable witnesses testify to having seen such things, although some hastily add that the same kind of controversy surrounds some qi gong exponents as Uri Geller attracts in the West. Television demonstrations by 'experts' who split bricks by projecting qi from their palms are less likely to be accepted. Those who have seen them will only say, 'Who can tell?'

Not surprisingly, there are fraudsters who achieve what appear to be amazing feats by sheer trickery, and fool the gullible into parting with their money, but the government is very harsh in its treatment of anyone caught offending in this way.

The power of the genuine qi gong masters is not in dispute, though they are few in number. Some are said to be able to 'see' the internal organs and to locate dysfunction merely by looking at a patient. Others are said to have powers of clairvoyance and to be able to look into the future. Healers can project their qi to perform miracle cures. One master, brought to the Traditional Medicine College in Canton to demonstrate to students, placed his hand below a stretcher on which an accident victim was lying, paralysed after his neck was broken, whereupon the injured man's limbs twitched into spasm.

Most TCM hospitals have qi gong doctors who practise by transmitting their qi to the patients. Watching them at work, white-coated and making a series of hand movements above an inert body on a couch, is a strange sight to Western eyes, but the patients they treat seem to derive benefit from it. The doctors will have qualified in all the other aspects of medical training, but have chosen to work in qi gong. They will treat everything from frozen shoulder to inoperable tumours. Many cases of cures through qi gong have been recorded, and although there are sceptical Chinese who will say that these are probably the result of the placebo effect, the genuine nature of the cure will not be in dispute. The *Nei Jing* states: 'Those who are habitually without disease help to train and adjust those who are sick. Therefore they train the patient to adjust his breathing and in order to train the patient, they act as an example.'

Any practice which has a long and venerable history becomes overlaid with a patina of magic, but the experts insist that there is nothing mysterious about qi gong. A master will go on practising it all his life and will still not have discovered the possibilities that lie within it. Yet a novice who learns the technique for health purposes is said to feel the benefit very quickly. Someone with hypertension, for example, who practises dutifully for three months, under medical guidance, will be able to take their blood pressure back to normal. However, there are certain dangers in the system. Anyone with a history of mental illness should not use qi gong, and it can have physical health hazards in other cases. Most teachers will ask pupils for details of their medical history before agreeing to take them on.

The South Kensington class with which this chapter began had been attending the course for a year. One pupil had come to try to cure a long-lasting back problem, another was seeking a cure for migraine. The only woman in the group had a cartilage problem in her knee, and she was convinced that the exercises were helping to cure it. An American businessman who enrolled because he thought that gentle breathing exercises and meditation would help to alleviate some of the stress of his fast-paced career, claimed it had changed his entire life. His change in outlook and health so impressed his wife that she too had enrolled to join the next session.

There are well-documented cases of cures achieved through the practice of qi gong, among them conditions like TB, migraine, stomach ulcers and diabetes. Even cancer patients are said to derive some benefit from exercises which aim to harness the qi with the will-power so that one becomes conscious of it, and able to clear blockages and direct it to areas of the body that are not functioning well.

People who have reached this stage describe the experience in many different ways. Most commonly, they claim that it feels like heat. Others experience it as flowing along the channels like a stream, or conveying a sense of lightness, tingling, weight, or even colour. Others practise for a year or more without reaching that stage, even though they will certainly derive considerable benefits from the discipline. Teachers say that the breakthrough will come to anyone who perseveres for three years.

Qi gong classes are becoming popular in Britain, but exponents of the art have yet to form themselves into any form of umbrella organization, with a set of professional standards to give the novice some indication of the quality of teaching he or she can expect to receive. In some cases, individual schools have set up their own associations, specifying their own standards, and these – though self-created – do give some guarantees and indication of quality.

The problem with all forms of complementary therapy is that no government body exists to register, control and regulate the practitioners. Anyone can set up a clinic or class offering any therapy they care to devise, provided they do not masquerade as a qualified doctor or make false claims.

As things stand, it is difficult for the interested Westerner to know where to locate teachers, or what their qualifications and particular form of qi gong may be. Britain has some extremely proficient qi gong masters, who have studied for years in their native land, often in styles passed down in the family. However, it is advisable to make detailed inquiries before enrolling.

A short list of practitioners can be found at the back of this book, though new classes are starting up every week all over the country. Finding the right teacher initially may be largely a matter of luck, but the more you learn about the system, the more you will be able to form your own opinions. A Chinese Grand Master in Beijing, asked about how and why his system worked, replied that some queries cannot be answered unless the questioner has a basic knowledge: 'First come inside, then ask questions,' he said. It is not customary to ask a teacher questions in China. One listens and learns. The Master will pass on his knowledge when he decides his pupil is ready to receive it. Ask a question before you have reached the level worthy to be answered, and it will simply be ignored, or the subject changed abruptly. However, a good teacher will be eager to outline the form of qi gong he follows, and to explain a little about the history behind it, and what it can do. An initial chat with the organizer will give some insight into his training methods, but speaking to members of the class will probably give a better idea of how it is run, and what benefits the students are experiencing. One of the characteristics of qi gong is that many teachers develop their own style, and there are often rivalries between the exponents of particular forms.

It is important to remember that this system is a deeply engrained part of Chinese culture, and therefore very much unknown territory to people in the West. Different systems will be good for sports training, physical fitness, meditation and health care. There is also a form of qi gong for sexual health and fitness.

In *Wild Swans*, Jung Chang's classic story recounting the fortunes of three generations of the women in her family, she writes about her grandmother's second husband, a TCM doctor who practised birth control through qi gong. He was able to reach orgasm without ejaculating. The jing energy, so vital to life, applies to the male sperm, the female ovum and menstrual cycle. A man who practises the right exercises can control and contain his semen. A woman will learn how to strengthen her sex organs. Together they can exchange their sexual energy to reach physical and spiritual ecstasy.

Classical qi gong systems

The Five Animal Frolics

This system is based on the movements of five animals – the bear, the bird, the tiger, deer and monkey. Hua Tuo said that the exercises would 'remove disease, strengthen the legs, produce sweating, increase the appetite and give a feeling of lightness.'

Muscle and Tendon-changing Classic and Bone Marrow-washing Classic

Da Mo was an Indian prince who came to China at the invitation of the Emperor during the Liang Dynasty (AD 502–57), fell out of favour at the Imperial Court and wisely withdrew to a monastery where he set to work to improve the health of the monks by living as a hermit for nine years. When he emerged, he had two classic systems to pass on to the sickly community. The Muscle and Tendon-changing Classic has been integrated into several martial arts for which the Shaolin Temple is still famous. The Bone Marrow-washing Classic uses the qi to clean the marrow in order to strengthen the immune system and nourish the brain to help it achieve enlightenment.

The Eight Pieces of Brocade

A celebrated soldier of the Southern Song Dynasty (AD 1127–1279), Marshal Yeuh Fei, trained his men in qi gong and is believed to have developed the hsing yi martial arts style. The Eight Pieces of Brocade was aimed at building up the body and maintaining health. In wars involving lengthy campaigns, the well-being of the fighting men was crucial. Battles were lost and won not just by military prowess, but by keeping epidemics at bay.

The Six Healing Sounds

During the Tang Dynasty (AD 618–907) Sun Si Miao wrote a book which contained 'The Song of Hygiene'. This involved Six Healing Sounds which use noise and posture to clear the energy channels.

Tai Qi Chuan

This blends the nei dan form of qi gong (internal system) with wei dan (external system). It is extremely popular in China.

Lulu Daoyin

Thought to be one of the earliest methods, stemming from a book written in 230 bc by Lu Tzu, entitled *The Spring and Autumn Annals*, in which he states that 'A long time ago, dancing was used to aid the flow of the qi and blood.' It involves spontaneous movement to music, with the qi moving the body at will.

CHAPTER TEN
Acupuncture

The World Health Organization endorses the use of acupuncture for:
Infections: colds, flu, bronchitis, hepatitis.
Internal: hypoglycaemia, asthma, high blood pressure, ulcers, colitis, indigestion, haemorrhoids, diarrhoea, constipation, diabetes.
Ear, nose and throat: deafness, tinnitus, dizziness, sinus infection, sore throat and hay fever.
Dermatological: eczema, acne, herpes.
Musculo-skeletal and neurologic: arthritis, neuralgia, sciatica, back pain, bursitis, tendonitis, stiff neck, Bell's palsy, headache, stroke, cerebral palsy, polio, sprains.
Mental-emotional: anxiety, depression, stress, insomnia.
Genito-urinary and reproductive: impotence, infertility, PMS, pelvic inflammatory disease, vaginitis, irregular periods, cramps.
Note: Acupuncture can occasionally induce an asthma attack in susceptible patients, and can cause premature labour in pregnant women.

Even the Chinese themselves have not yet ascertained precisely how acupuncture and moxibustion work. No one can say exactly how the discovery was made, or when needles were first used in medical treatment, but it goes far beyond the time of recorded history. For a treatment to have been in use for almost as long as mankind itself, and yet still to retain some of its mystery, makes it doubly remarkable. Unfortunately, it also means that it is still regarded by many doctors in the West as a placebo.

Sufferers who have found pain relief or cure from acupuncture, however, know that in such cases a placebo is merely a cure by another name. People who have had acupuncture at the hands of a practitioner skilled in TCM know that the experience is not 'all in the mind'. They can explain internal sensations directly connected with the action of a needle at a particular point, even though they know nothing about the theory of acupuncture. Researchers have recorded the following physical sensations produced by the needles: numbness, distension, warmth, heaviness, tenseness, coldness or burning and sometimes a feeling radiating along the length of the channel.

We still tend to associate acupuncture with pain relief, for which it is indeed very effective, but in China it has far wider uses, not just in curing disease and mental disorders, but also in controlling epidemics. Sir Winston Churchill on a visit to China reported seeing a patient in the burns unit of a Shanghai hospital who was able to walk after acupuncture treatment, despite the fact that 94 per cent of his body was damaged by third-degree burns. When he told British doctors about this on his return, he was assured that no patient could possibly survive with over 75 per cent of burns on his body.

Moxibustion, which simply means applying heat by burning a twist of moxa wool (the dried leaves of the artemisia plant) on the end of the needle, is used as an extra stimulant to impel the body to provide energy to assist the healing process. In TCM terminology, acupuncture and moxa work by:

- Reducing what is excessive (alleviating headaches)
- Increasing what is deficient (treating asthma)
- Cooling what is hot (soothing eczema)
- Moving what is stagnant (shrinking benign tumours)
- Stabilizing what is reckless (stopping nose-bleeds)
- Raising what is falling (correcting prolapse)
- Lowering what is rising (controlling high blood pressure)
- Strengthening the resistance (inflammation)
- Eliminating the pathogenic agents (curing colds and flu)

The Chinese, who have carried out more research into acupuncture than any other nation, have proved that it has analgesic effects. A respected Beijing neurophysiologist, Professor Jia Hing Han, established the neurochemical basis of pain relief. Research teams have produced evidence that it can stimulate endorphins in the brain which produce clinical analgesia; it can stimulate the adrenal gland to produce its own cortisone. Experiments have demonstrated that acupuncture can bring about changes of functional activity in the hypothalamus-pituitary-adrenal system, and alter the composition of the blood.

The fact that acupuncture took pain away and cured sickness confirmed to the early medicine men their theory that the outside of the body directly affected and influenced the internal condition. The two are connected by invisible pathways which lie beneath the surface of the skin, and circulate in a continuous loop of main channels and interconnecting collaterals linking the organs and the viscera, which are called in Chinese the jinglao.

There are thirty-five channels in all. Twelve main channels are connected with the lungs, the large intestine, the stomach, spleen, heart, small intestine, urinary bladder, kidney, pericardium, the sanjiao (the abstract organ often translated as the 'triple burner', which is thought to mean the endocrine gland), the gallbladder and the liver.

These twelve channels run along the limbs, the trunk and the head, and are in pairs, at the right- and left-hand side of the body. Two others run vertically up the middle of the body, one at the back, one at the front, and are called the 'conception' and the 'governor' channels. They do not connect particular organs, but they are the only remaining channels with acupoints running along them.

The twelve major channels have superficial pathways under the surface of the skin, and deep pathways internally. Smaller channels called collaterals link one with another, so that they form a continuous circle around the frame. After these come the Eight Miraculous Channels, which act as a sort of back-up system. They have a reserve pool of energy so that they can either supply a deficiency or take up any excess. These are paired, and include the conception and governor channels. The others are the thrusting and girdle channels.

The thrusting channel runs deep inside the centre of the body from the perineum to the crown. It contains 'cauldrons' located at more or less the same acupoints as those on the surface at the governor and conception channels. The cauldrons are storage vessels where the qi is more apparent.

The girdle is the only channel which runs horizontally. As the name suggests, it encircles the waist like a belt. The other four, called the yin wei mo and the yang wei mo, the yin qiao mo and the yang qiao mo, connect and link the limbs with the internal organs.

Next are the junction channels, fifteen in all. Fourteen of these have an interconnecting function linking each of the main channels and the eight extra meridians, and connect yin and yang. The remaining channel is known as the 'great envelope of the spleen', which is located under the armpit on the side of the chest. It joins everything together.

These are the pathways along which qi travels, assisting the blood and body fluids, maintaining the correct balance between yin and yang, and protecting the body against disease. Traditionally, there are 365 points on the skin which directly connect with the vital organs, and where the qi can be stimulated by the insertion of needles. Recent research has identified many more, and modern-day acupuncture charts show over 2,000, but the traditional points still tend to be the ones practitioners use.

Modern needles are extremely finely made precision instruments. Electro-acupuncture is another modern refinement. A small box with a probe attached emits a buzzing signal at an acupoint, and gives objective readings, enabling the patient to be tested before and after each session.

No matter what technology can reveal about needling, the traditional doctors use it the way their forefathers did. The fingers of a skilled teacher are the most sensitive instrument there is, and since the doctor's own qi is involved in the treatment, no machine can ever equal that. Some doctors practise acupressure, which uses the same points on the body as acupuncture but with the pressure being applied with the doctor's fingers rather than needles. This treatment, often combined with massage, is highly effective for skeletal, muscle and ligament problems, and is useful for patients who are nervous of needles.

To TCM doctors, the organs of the body are not important anatomically, it is their functions that matter, and these are influenced by the element associated with them. All disease is the result of disharmony. For further details on the organs of the body in TCM, see Chapter 3.

The heart governs the blood and is open to the tongue, its element is fire, and it houses the spirit. Therefore, disharmony in the heart will not be confined to a cardiac complaint, as it would be in Western medicine. It could be involved with a speech impediment, or an emotional condition such as manic depression, as well as a simple problem such as chilblains caused through poor circulation. Any of these complaints, and a number of others, would be treated along the heart channel.

The lungs govern breath and are open to the nose. Their element is metal and they rule over the skin. They also receive the 'heavenly qi', which is both the air which we breathe and the spiritual quality which gives meaning and purpose to life. Disharmony here can affect the sinuses, the throat and the chest, or create an emotional problem whereby the victim becomes apathetic and lethargic, and loses interest in his or her surroundings.

The liver governs the movement of qi and is open to the eyes. Its element is wood, and it rules over the eyes. Most menstrual disorders are treated through the liver channel, as are eye problems such as conjunctivitis, and any stress disorders associated with anger, which is the emotion linked with the liver.

The spleen is the centre of the body, connected with the functions of the other organs like the axle of a wheel. It transforms food and drink into qi and blood and distributes them around the body. It rules over the muscles. Dysfunctions associated with it are digestive problems and prolapse.

The kidneys have a very special function in TCM theory. They store the essence of life. They are open to the ears, and their element is water, which in medical terms means not just urine, but also seminal and hormonal fluids. The adrenal glands which are just above the kidneys (and in Western medicine, anatomically distinct from them) are regarded in TCM as an integral part of the kidney function. The kidneys also rule over the bones and the marrow, which nourishes the brain. Water retention, infertility problems, deafness and tinnitus are all regarded as dysfunctions which can be treated via the kidney channel.

The names of each of the acupoints on the channels give an inkling of their function. The spirit path, on the heart channel, is self-explanatory. The gate of hope on the liver channel points to its function as the organ which gives a sense of direction and optimism, when it is working harmoniously. The spleen has an acupoint called earth motivator, which can help to reinvigorate people with a tendency to brood or think too deeply. An acupoint called bubbling spring is sited on the kidney channel. The kidneys, receptacles of inheritance and sexual energy, are the organs which irrigate the body.

The channels of the zang organs have a storage function, and are therefore yin. The fu-organs, the viscera, are all yang, because they are hollow and act as processors. All have their own particular functions, though each is closely linked with a primary organ. One of them has a particular responsibility.

The channel of the pericardium (the fibrous sheath that surrounds the heart) is known as the heart's 'protector'. The heart, as the emperor of the body, is vital to the smooth running of the state. It is therefore vulnerable to attack and to pressure, and needs a guard to watch over it. The pericardium fulfils that function. Its channel is often more effective in treating cardiac conditions than the heart channel itself. It also has an emotional function, because, just as we do in the West, the Chinese believe the heart is the seat of the feelings.

The pericardium's job is to protect the heart from emotional damage, and since love is inextricably linked with sex, the psychological interplay of boy-meets-girl comes within the remit of the pericardium. Some sexual dysfunctions and relationship difficulties causing emotional illness would be treated on this channel.

The large intestine is linked to the lungs, and part of its function is to discharge waste material through the bowels, and toxins through the skin. This channel will be used to treat constipation and diarrhoea, skin problems or sinus trouble.

The small intestine is paired with the heart. It is responsible for 'receiving and making things thrive', which, because of its close functional proximity to the heart, it does for the mind and spirit as well as the digestive system. It ends at a point in front of the ear, and is also used in the treatment of some hearing disorders.

The gallbladder is connected to the liver, and in TCM it is believed to be connected with a person's self-image and personal confidence. The shrinking violet personality, the Chinese would say, has a 'small gallbladder'. This channel is used to treat menstrual difficulties, eye problems, headaches, arthritic hips and knees, and lack of confidence or indecision.

The triple burner isn't, strictly speaking, an organ at all. It is the body's thermostat, although it has its own channel because it is closely connected with the other eleven organs. In TCM theory, the trunk of the body is divided into three sections, all of which control the heat within it; and are responsible for assuring that the same even temperature is maintained throughout the body.

The upper burner is located in the chest, the middle lies between the diaphragm and the navel, and the lower burner is in the lower abdomen. The three work as one, and their function is to balance the internal yin and yang, and the fire and water. When the weather turns cold, it is the triple burner which adjusts the body temperature to adapt to the changing climate. If there is a dysfunction affecting the triple burner, a chill or fever will be the result. Too much yang, for example, will cause the body to overheat or will dry up some of the body fluids. Too much yin will have the opposite effect. This is the channel which will be worked on in illnesses characterized by a high temperature, or severe chills.

The stomach channel sends the food to the spleen and is regarded as the keeper of the storehouse and granaries. It begins the digestive process and will be the channel used in some gastric disorders and bowel problems. Because food has such profound psychological influences, it is also the channel involved in treatment for eating disorders.

The bladder channel is closely connected with the kidney and its main function is to distribute the fluids in the body, getting rid of 'bad' water. The channel runs the length of the body, beginning at the corner of the eye, crossing the head, and passing twice down the back before running right down the leg to end at the little toe. It acts on many skeletal problems, sciatica, many types of back pain, and also on cystitis or incontinence.

The encircling qi

The body's biorhythms are a comparatively new concept in the Western world, but it has existed in China for centuries. The Chinese count the day and night together, not as twenty-four hours, but as twelve. Each one of their hours is equal to two of ours. There are twelve hours in the day, and twelve major organs in the body, through which the qi flows constantly, but it reaches a peak in each organ for one hour of the Chinese day.

This is consistent with the notion of man as a small cosmos, and it bears out the biological reality of energy movement within the body. Between 11 a.m. and 1 pm it is at its peak in the heart; it then goes into the small intestine from 1 pm until 3 pm. It is in the bladder from 3 pm to 5 pm; in the kidneys from 5 pm to 7 pm; in the pericardium from 7 pm to 9 pm; in the triple burner from 9 pm to 11 pm; in the gallbladder from 11 pm to 1 am; in the liver from 1 am to 3 am; in the lungs from 3 am to 5 am; in the large intestine from 5 am to 7 am; in the stomach from 7 am to 9 am; and in the spleen from 9 am to 11 am. It has therefore revolved around the body in the same way as the earth revolves around the sun, and of course each organ has a point at the opposite end of the cycle when the qi is at its weakest.

Qi also completes one cycle up the back and front of the body, in the governor and conception channels, hence the female menstrual cycle. It is at its peak at the top of the head during the full moon, and at the new moon (the Chinese refer to it as the 'empty' moon) it is in the perineum.

The qi also has a seasonal flow throughout the year. It reaches its peak in the liver and gallbladder in the spring, in the heart and small intestine (and the triple burner and pericardium) in summer, in the stomach and the spleen in Indian summer, in the lungs and large intestine in autumn, and in the kidneys and bladder in the winter.

The twelve major channels

Lung: Starts 5 cm/2 inches from the nipple and runs in the direction of the arm, ending in the thumb. Line for asthma, coughs, chest and shoulder pain.

Large intestine: Starts at the tip of the index finger, runs up the arm, over the shoulder to the opposite side of the nose. Line for head, face, mouth, neck and throat pain, lower jaw and teeth problems.

Stomach: Starts underneath the eye, down the side of the body and leg to the second toe. Line for digestive disorders, ulcers, mouth problems, high fever and diarrhoea.

Spleen: Starts at the big toe, runs up the centre front of leg through the side of the abdomen and curves to the side of the rib-cage. Line for menstrual problems, stomach trouble and blood deficiencies.

Pericardium: Starts from the nipple up to the shoulder and down the arm to the middle finger. Line for chest pains, heart problems, palpitations, all forms of sickness.

Triple burner: Starts at the ring finger, runs up the back of the arm and side of the neck to the temple. Line for nervous problems, paralysis, tinnitus, migraine, neuralgia.

Gallbladder: Starts at the outer edge of the eye, runs zig-zag over the trunk, down the side of the leg to the fourth toe. Line for pain at the side of the head, back and joints, thigh, knee, and leg, also malaria.

Liver: Starts at the big toe and goes up to the outside of the rib-cage under the nipple. Line for hernia, chest stuffiness, lumbago and menstrual problems.

Heart: Starts at the armpit and runs down to the little finger. Line for insomnia, poor memory, lack of concentration and mental problems such as epilepsy and schizophrenia.

Small intestine: Starts at the little finger, goes up the arm, across the shoulder to the ear. Line for jaw, neck, shoulder and arm pain and for frequent urination.

Bladder: Starts at the inside corner of the eye, goes over the head, down the back and leg to the little toe. All the shu points, the 'sources of energy', run down this channel.

Kidney: Begins on the sole of the foot, runs to just below the collarbone. Line for genital diseases, bladder and kidney complaints, breathlessness, cataracts and blurred vision.

The two unpaired meridians

Conception vessel: Runs from deep inside the lower abdomen, up the centre of the body to the root of the tongue.

Governor vessel: Starts from deep inside the lower abdomen, up the back, over the head and ends under the lip on the upper jaw.

CHAPTER ELEVEN
Gynaecology

A familiar sight at the Outpatients Clinic in the Gynaecology Department of a TCM hospital, is a row of young women, each lying with a small, smoking box on her abdomen. They are having moxibustion treatment for painful periods, and it works.

In the West, there are two familiar and all-encompassing remedies for gynaecological problems: hormone therapy or surgery, neither of which is free from controversy.

Many women who have had their lives transformed by hormone replacement therapy are firm advocates of its use, but medical opinion is still divided on the long-term effects of the progesterone and oestrogen in HRT. There are similar concerns about the contraceptive pill, and debate continues over radical surgery in cases of breast cancer and uterine disorders.

In China, women automatically have a third choice if they experience gynaecological illness: treatment with traditional herbs and acupuncture. The results are often very successful. Pre-menstrual tension, menopausal symptoms, pelvic inflammation and threatened miscarriage are all treated using herbs as the main therapy.

Foot massage is another well-regarded remedy for painful periods. Every acupoint is found in the feet, and TCM regards the relation of the feet to the body as like that of the root to the tree. Treat the root and the tree will flourish.

Health care for women in large cities in China includes an annual pap smear to check for early indications of cervical cancer. If pre-cancerous cells are detected, they will be treated by a combination of Western and TCM therapies. The herbal medicine will help healthy new tissue to grow, and is applied direct to the cervix.

Where the condition is in the early, CIN 1 stage, the herbal applications usually restore the cervical cells to normal within a week. In CIN 2 cases, the condition will take between two and four weeks to treat, and at the CIN 3 stage, although more intensive treatment is required, and patient response is slower, doctors say that their approach, which is to correct a spleen deficiency, and clear away dampness and heat, will in most cases strengthen the immune system and result in a complete cure.

Gynaecologists in TCM hospitals also often give treatment via the ear, which, like the foot, contains every acupoint in the body. A variety of menstrual problems are treated by inserting a tiny seed called wang bu liu xing zi into the earlobe, which patients are instructed to press four or five times a day. In Western terms, this has the effect of regulating the endocrinal function. In TCM, it strengthens the kidney and the lung. TCM doctors in Britain often offer the same treatment, although they use a plastic replica of the seed, rather than the real thing. It fits comfortably in the ear at the appropriate acupoint, and can be left in place for several days. The seeds are also used in other treatments, for example to help smokers who are trying to give up tobacco.

Acupuncture can clear certain cases of blocked fallopian tubes. It can be effective against polycystic ovaries, although the treatment involves intensive needling and recovery is slow.

Women with small fibroids detected at an early stage will be treated in a Chinese hospital with powerful herbal medicines which can dissolve them without the need for surgery. Larger fibroids still have to be surgically removed, but they will be shrunk first, requiring a less drastic operation. Some doctors use acupuncture to produce the same result. If a fibroid is not deeply embedded in the uterine wall, acupuncture is often successful.

Fibroids are considered to be the result of cold in the uterus caused through poor diet and environmental cold. A TCM practitioner will advise women who are vegetarians to be wary of eating too many raw foods. Food items which are cold in nature, such as fruit and most leaf vegetables, especially cabbage, can contribute to internal cold.

In Tianjin First Teaching Hospital, gynaecologists had treated 800 cases of hystermyoma (tumour of the uterus) with a mixture of Western and TCM therapies. Treatment lasted for three months, but the department head reported that the outcome was successful in 98 per cent of the cases.

Chinese physicians believe that a lot of gynaecological problems are connected to the blood, often caused by liver qi stagnation and heavily influenced by emotional factors and by diet. The irritability that often accompanies the menopause, and the mood swings and weepiness that characterize PMT, can all be traced back to the liver, the organ which influences the emotional state. There is a second factor, for the liver meridian is the main channel with major collaterals passing through the uterus and ovaries.

Pre-menstrual tension results when the blood is channelled downwards to the uterus, causing the liver blood to become deficient and affect the heart, producing 'empty heart fire'. This can also cause insomnia, since the spirit resides in the mind during the day, and the heart at night. If the heart is troubled by fire, the spirit is disturbed and cannot rest. PMT which manifests itself in severe diarrhoea and vomiting, by contrast, is caused by a spleen and kidney condition, since both those organs are involved in the production of blood.

In TCM, the adrenal gland, which secretes the body's natural hormones, and is connected to the central nervous system, is included with the kidneys. The two kidneys are considered to have separate functions in TCM, the right for water and the left for fire. The water element includes hormonal secretions, and the fire element involves the source of vitality, of heat energy, in the body.

Dysmenorrhoea is the result of a deficiency of the kidney and spleen, and where there is pain before and after a period, indications are that an energy deficiency has resulted in blood stagnation. The patient may also suffer from a liver blood deficiency which can cause severe migraine. There is a well-known patented tablet which is very effective in cases of period problems called Women's Precious Pills and these can now be bought in Britain in some Chinese herbal clinics.

The case of a nursing sister who suffered years of misery from gynaecological complaints before being cured by TCM neatly illustrates the holistic approach of traditional medicine. Stephanie was born in Malaya, and in 1966 came to England where she qualified as a midwife. When she married and settled in rural Surrey she began to have problems with interim bleeding, and two D&C operations failed to clear the problem.

She was then diagnosed as suffering from a Batholin cyst and polyps in the uterus, which resulted in severe pain before and after a period. Investigations were made in hospital and small fibroids were also discovered. At the same time, she developed conjunctivitis, and was referred to an eye specialist who prescribed hydrocortisone. The eye treatment helped in the short term, but the following month, the conjunctivitis flared up again.

Stephanie had switched to night duty at the hospital so that she could be with her young son during the day, and was feeling tired and stressed in addition to the physical problems she was suffering. Her period pains were now so bad that she was prescribed a very strong and effective painkiller.

As a nurse, Stephanie was aware of the side-effects which can sometimes arise from prolonged use of that particular drug. It can accumulate in the liver and, if taken in excess, has been thought to cause aplastic anaemia. She decided against taking it, and continued to try to cope. By now, hospital tests showed that her ovaries had swollen to ten times their normal size, and her uterus was the same size as at three months in pregnancy. Tests showed no malignancy, but there was an overgrowth of tissue, so a radical hysterectomy was performed, and Stephanie was given an implant of HRT. Two years of good health followed before menopausal symptoms appeared, the conjunctivitis flared up again, and a lump appeared in her breast. It was asperated, but three more followed. The doctor could not discover the cause of the problem, or how to treat it. 'You may just have to learn to live with it,' she was told.

Coming from a Chinese family, Stephanie was familiar with traditional medicine, and decided that if the conventional system could not help her, perhaps TCM could. Benefiting from her own medical background, she decided not merely to seek TCM treatment, but to study the system to see if she could help herself to understand her increasing physical problems. She enrolled at a London postgraduate school run by a practitioner who was trained in Western medicine as well as TCM, and who now taught Western doctors and health professionals.

Stephanie's medical history provided a first study case for the students. Her face was swollen, her tongue had a blue tinge to it, and she suffered from profuse sweating and sleeplessness. The various symptoms, the conjunctivitis and the gynaecological complaints, were not regarded as separate ailments, but were all manifestations of the same dysfunction.

The main cause was liver stagnation with congealed blood and a total depletion of yang energy. In TCM, the liver is connected with the eyes, which explained the conjunctivitis. Previously, Stephanie had wondered whether the conjunctivitis and swollen face were the result of living near a large wood where the summer air was often filled with pollen. Now she was being taught to recognize all the symptoms as stemming from a single source. Acupuncture was given to clear the liver channel; she had a course of moxa to tonify the yang energy, and herbal tablets to tonify the liver yin and kidney yang.

Within weeks the dampness in her body had cleared, her sleep pattern improved and the sweating had stopped. As the months went by, the breast lumps disappeared too. A year later, the pupil/ patient is still working as a midwife, and continuing her studies into TCM. Like the principal of her college, she values the merits of both systems of medicine, and looks forward to the day when the best of both can be combined.

CHAPTER TWELVE
In the Medicine Cabinet

Patent medicines are just as much part of everyday life for the Chinese as they are for people in Britain. Tablets with names such as Women's Precious Pills, mentioned in the previous chapter, the Free and Easy Wanderer and the Six Gentlemen are famous throughout the mainland.

Some resulted from old prescriptions, closely guarded secrets passed down through the generations, and originally made only in one family firm. When Chairman Mao decided that the benefits of TCM should become more widely available for all, the owners were persuaded to divulge the formulae for mass-production.

As everyone knew, revealing the ingredients was only part of the story. The right and the particular refinements of preparation could make subtle differences to the curative qualities of the pills. So although some of the famous prescriptions are now produced by pharmaceutical companies all over China, and those sold by Chinese herbalists in Britain will all have passed the quality control of the People's Republic, some brands may be just a little more effective than others, because they are still produced by the family or firm who owned the original prescription. The uninitiated have to trust to luck, although a statement on the packaging that the company has been awarded a government medal for their product is a useful pointer. A few of the remedies listed below contain animal products, and where this is the case, the particular ingredient – antelope horn or gecko, for example – is mentioned. None contains prohibited or endangered species. Those who do not wish to use anything involving animals can choose from alternatives which are purely herbal in content.

These tablets, though readily available throughout mainland China and Hong Kong, are not as yet on general sale in the UK. They can be obtained through TCM doctors and traditional Chinese pharmacists, who will advise on the type likely to help. Anyone who suffers from a serious condition should always consult their own GP before taking any other medicine, but for common ailments which are not serious, or for conditions where allopathic remedies are not proving effective, these long-established remedies may prove helpful. They have been tried and tested in their country of origin for decades, if not centuries, and are universally available in China, where their curative qualities are known throughout the country.

Anorexia
Xiang Sha Liu Jun Zi Wan (Six Noble Ingredients) For the treatment of indigestion, anorexia, abdominal distension, peptic ulcer, chronic gastritis. Contains bighead atractylodes rhizome, poria, liquorice, tangerine peel, pinellia tuber; plus costas root and amomum fruit.

Arthritis
Du Hou Ji Sheng Wan Considered very effective in clearing wind damp and cold from the body. Taken for back pain, knee pain and arthritis which is affected by cold weather.

Asthma
Ge Jie Dingchuan Wan Said to nourish yin, clear away lung heat and relieve coughing. Contains animal products, including gecko, which is very effective in asthma treatment and in common use in TCM hospitals; also the shell of freshwater turtle.
Zhisou Dingchuan Gao Contains radish extract, pear extract, fresh ginger and ephedra.
Runfei Gao Lung-nourishing semifluid extract for asthma, also chest congestion (specially recommended for the old and weak). Contains pear extract, pilose asiabell root, astragalus root, root of tatarian aster.

Back pain (lumbago)
Lui Wei Di Huang Wan (Six Rehmannia Pills) A well-known remedy which is said to nourish the kidney and treat liver deficiency. As well as easing lumbago, it is helpful for tinnitus, heavy sweating and dizziness, and is also used in cases of low sperm count and diabetes.

Influenza, colds and sore throats
Yin Qiao Jie Du Pian Colds with fever, headache, cough, dry mouth and sore throat. Contains honeysuckle flower, arctium fruit, forsythia fruit, platycodon root, peppermint, lophantherum, schizonepeta spike, liquorice and fermented soybean.
Zhong Gan Ling For colds which are caused by a chill and include runny nose and sneezing but no fever.
Fanggan Pian Prevents the common cold and strengthens resistance to chronic bronchitis. Contains astragalus root.

Tianjin Ganmao Pian For influenza. Contains arctium fruit, forsythia and honeysuckle, prepared soybean, platycodon root.

Cough
Chuan Bei Bi Pa Lu A very effective linctus which can treat all ages.

Colitis
Shen Ling Bai Zhu Wan The pills help the spleen and clear 'dampness' from the body. Treats colitis, loose stools, diarrhoea, sickness and nausea, and poor digestion.

Diabetes
Yuquan Wan Treatment to relieve thirst, clear away heat, arrest irritability and nourish yin and kidney. It does not cure diabetes, but it will alleviate some of the symptoms. Contains peuraria root, snake gourd root, dried rehmannia root. As diabetes is a serious condition, it is especially important to consult your GP before taking any other medicines.

Emotional problems
Giupi Wan (Return Spleen Tablets) A favourite and long-established remedy found in every Chinese household. It acts to tonify the spleen and nourish the blood. Taken for anaemia, heavy periods, insomnia, palpitations, dizziness and poor digestion.
Tian Wang Bu Xin Dan (Celestial Emperor) Used for the relief of palpitations, insomnia, restlessness, poor memory and lack ol concentration. Also useful to treat constipation in the elderly.

General debility
Liu Jun Zi Wan (Six Gentlemen) Sometimes translated as the 'noble ingredients' (see under Anorexia above), this prescription contains half a dozen herbs highly prized for their curative qualities in a variety of ailments. The pills are a favourite remedy throughout China as a reliable pick-me-up for those who feel generally run down, or suffer trom poor appetite, sickness or mucus and phlegm.

Geriatric conditions
Qingchunbao Pian For general debility in advanced age and deficiency following illness. Contains ginseng and ophiopogon root.

Gynaecological complaints

Ba Zhen Wan (Women's Precious Pills) This is a great standby in any family medicine cupboard in mainland China. As the name suggests, the most common use is for menstrual problems such as dysmenorrhoea, PMT and menopausal symptoms. The pills' effectiveness lies in treating general weakness of qi and blood, so they can also be taken by men, and are helpful in cases of anaemia and general fatigue.

Wu Ji Bai Feng Wan (Black Chicken and White Phoenix Pills) For period pains, leucorrhea and irregular periods.

Zhe Bai Di Huang Wan (Six Rehmannia Pills Plus Two) Recommended for the treatment of hot flushes, restlessness and night sweats.

Buxue Ningshen Pian For insomnia, frequent urination, irregular menstruation, soreness and weakness in the loins and knees. Contains fleece-flower stem, spatholobus stem, prepared rehmannia root.

Dang Gui Jing Pian Helpful in regulating the periods and for treating irregular menstruation accompanied by headaches and constipation. Also relieves menstrual pain. Contains Chinese angelica root.

Fu Ke Shi Wei Pian For irregular menstruation and dysmenorrhoea. Contains Chinese angelica root, red peony root, corydalis tuber, nutgrass flatsedge rhizome.

Jin Hi Chongji For treatment of endometriosis, pelvic inflammation. Contains infusion of cherokee rose and spatholobus stem.

Nu Bao For regulating menstruation, stopping irregular bleeding, leucorrhoea, sterility due to cold in the womb and abdominal pain after delivery.

Xiao Yan Wan (The Free and Easy Wanderer) This is a familiar remedy for Chinese women. It works by soothing the liver, which is the main channel for the treatment of menstrual problems and other gynaecological conditions. The pills are good for menopausal symptoms, PMT, depression, migraine headaches and irregular menstruation. This well-known prescription also relieves stagnation of qi energy. It has been in use for generations.

High blood pressure

Qi Ju Di Huang Wan (Six Rehmannia Pills Plus Two) Six Rehmannia Pills is an old and revered remedy, to which herbal doctors add an extra ingredient or two for particular ailments. This prescription treats liver, kidney and yin deficiencies, and is used in cases of vertigo, poor vision, cataracts and tinnitus, as well as high blood pressure. It is especially important that people suffering from HBP always seek treatment from their GP.

Incontinence
Jin Suo Gu Jing Wan (Golden Lock Tea) Aptly named preparation which helps control bladder weakness, spontaneous sweating, emission and chronic leucorrhoea.

Low sperm count
Lui Wei Di Huang Wan (Six Rehmannia Pills) In China, this is a well-known prescription which treats a variety of conditions. It is said to increase the sperm count.

Prolapse
Bu Zhong Yi Qi Wan (Centre Qi Boosting Pills) Helpful in cases of prolapse of the uterus or kidneys, and also used for chronic diarrhoea, and to treat tiredness, fatigue, and poor digestion.

Sports injuries
Die Da Wan Hua You (Oil) Good for treating bad bruising, burns, old injuries and cuts, and for the relief of pain in arthritis.
Shang Shi Zhi Ton Gao (Plaster for external use) For pain relief in cases of sport injuries, also lumbago, sciatica and arthritis.

Stomach upsets
Huo Xiang Zheng Qi Yuan For stomach chills with diarrhoea and sickness, also for tummy bugs and food poisoning.

Throat infections
Niuhuang Yijin Pian For acute and chronic pharyngitis, laryngitis. Contains phellodendron bark and artificial cow-bezoar.
Yanlixiao Jiaonang For relief in cases of swollen sore throat, upper respiratory tract infection, acute or chronic tonsillitis, also dysentery and diarrhoea. Can also be used to treat the common cold.

CHAPTER THIRTEEN
A–Z

Abscess

Caused by bacterial infection under the skin, abcesses are usually considered a heat and fire poison in the blood. Treatment is given to clear the heat, reduce the fire and eliminate poison from the body. Commonly used herbs include Chinese golden thread, dandelion or wild chrysanthemum and violet, made into herbal tea. Applications of external medicine, using rhubarb or peony flowers, ground up and mixed with sesame oil, will help to hasten the healing process.

Acid stomach

The term covers a variety of conditions, but usually describes the regurgitation of acid or heartburn caused by indigestion. In TCM, spleen deficiency and an imbalance of spleen and liver are regarded as the main causes. The doctor will give treatment to tonify the spleen, to dry 'dampness' and soothe the liver, reducing stagnation. Herbs used include ginseng, poria and liquorice; orange peel and eggshell are also used. The patient will be advised about a diet to avoid acidic food or 'cold' food, reducing stagnation. Western doctors also recommend care with the diet, eating small, regular meals based mainly on bland foods such as chicken, rice, milk and fish. Fried and fatty foods should be avoided.

Acne

One of the most common problems for young people, especially during adolescence. Boys suffer more than girls, but occasionally the complaint persists beyond the teenage years. Western medicine considers this a hormone imbalance. TCM regards it as a problem of damp heat which is brought about either by overeating hot and damp food, or as the result of the digestive system being imbalanced. This means that the spleen and stomach are not functioning adequately, and occasionally the trouble can be traced to the lungs.

Teenage acne usually clears up itself, but those who have a problem with it should avoid deep-fried food like fish and chips or crisps, or hot foods like chilli and curry. They should drink very little alcohol, and cut down on chocolate.

Severe or chronic acne can be treated with antibiotics by a Western doctor, but if it persists, a TCM doctor will investigate the action of the spleen and stomach and use purging herbs such as rhubarb to open the bowels. The doctor will also give herbs to purify the blood and will recommend a special diet. It is better not to put too many external preparations on the spots. Smothering them in oils and lotions will only make matters worse.

AIDS

AIDS is a new disease to Chinese medicine but immune system deficiencies are not new; they have existed for centuries, and TCM doctors and clinics in Britain and America have been treating patients with some small success. In Chinese medicine, AIDS is considered a weakness of the kidneys and the spleen, mainly caused by a self-indulgent lifestyle, especially drinking to excess. TCM is unequivocal on the topic of moderation. Any excess, emotional or physical, will harm the body. The jing energy, the very essence of life held by the kidney, is injured by excess. Lifestyle is therefore crucial to well-being, and sexual promiscuity, or drug abuse, will inevitably lead to health problems.

Drug abuse weakens the system and causes kidney yin deficiency, with symptoms such as night fever and coughs. Combined damp heat then invades the body. In TCM treatment is mainly given to nourish the kidneys and strengthen the spleen. TCM doctors in the Western world treat AIDS with a combination of herbs, among them astragalus, Chinese snake gourd and Six Rehmmania Pills or Return Spleen Pills. They are able to bolster the immune system to prevent complications and prolong life, preventing HIV from turning into AIDS. A chemical extract from the Chinese snake gourd, which looks rather like a cucumber, is perhaps the most promising drug produced so far in the race against the advance of this terrible disease. It is undergoing trials with the American Food and Drugs Administration, and if it fulfills its early promise, we may be nearing the day when a cure is discovered.

In ancient times, the Chinese snake gourd was used to procure abortions, although no one knew how it worked. A Hong Kong scientist, Professor Yeung, carrying out research into its action, discovered that it selectively kills the trophoblast cell, which regulates activity of the placenta. The herb also targets cells in the body called macrophages (scavenger cells which clean up stray toxins). In America, Dr Michael McGrath, director of an AIDS research laboratory in San Francisco, found that some macrophages can be infected by the HIV virus. This was another step forward in understanding why none of the medicines so far produced has proved to be a cure. They killed infected T-cells, but not infected macrophages. The extract trichosanthin, which Professor Yeung's team at the Chinese University had isolated from the Chinese snake gourd, apparently kills infected cells in the body's immune system, but leaves the healthy cells alone. He sent a small phial to Dr McGrath, who carried out trials on volunteers.

Research is still going on into a number of individual herbs, but Chinese doctors strongly believe that the best approach is to continue to treat the whole system, and that the interaction between a combination of herbs will always prove more effective than extracts alone.

Alcoholism

Consumed in large quantities, alcohol is a poison which destroys brain cells, and can adversely affect every organ in the body. Social drinking can turn into a physical dependence on alcohol so gradually that family and friends may have difficulty in persuading the alcoholic that he or she has a problem. Once the addiction develops, the body can become so dependent upon alcohol that it is unable to function without it. Symptoms include depression, memory blackouts and hallucinations.

The diagnosis in TCM is that excessive alcohol consumption causes too much heat in the body, damaging the liver and stomach. Herbs would be first used to take the heat out of the liver and the blood. In mild cases, strong green tea is used as a cooling agent. Chronic alcoholism would involve using kudzu vine or watermelon to detoxify the blood.

Treatment to alleviate the physical damage will help, but alcoholism usually has a psychological cause and the patient would be advised to seek counselling and to join a self-help group.

Amnesia

Temporary memory loss can be caused by severe shock often following an accident, and sometimes illness. Meningitis, epilepsy or brain tumour can trigger amnesia. It is considered a kidney weakness, so the 'essence' of the kidney is toned with the eucommia bark, wolfberry seed, mulberry fruit or dodder seed. Once the function of the kidney has been strengthened, it will nourish the brain, improving the memory. A common Chinese saying is that 'kidneys nourish the marrow and marrow feeds the brain'.

Anaemia

A variety of illnesses come under the general term anaemia, the commonest of which results from an iron deficiency. Pernicious anaemia is caused by the body's failure to absorb adequate quantities of vitamin B12, and it can affect vegans whose diet may lack protein. Megaloblastic anaemia is caused by a deficiency of folic acid found in fresh vegetables and liver.

Chinese medicine regards anaemia as resulting from the spleen not transforming qi correctly. A herbal remedy widely used to treat iron deficiency anaemia in mainland China is called Return Spleen Tablets (giupi wan in Chinese). Chinese medicine acknowledges that anaemia is the result of an iron deficiency, but where Western doctors might prescribe iron supplements, the view in TCM is that the body gets all the iron it requires from a properly balanced diet, therefore a doctor's first concern must be to restore its own ability to absorb the iron effectively, by restoring the function of the spleen.

A similar method of treatment can also be helpful for women who suffer from sickness or constipation through taking iron supplements during pregnancy, as it does not cause the side-effect of constipation. The herbs used enable the body to absorb and maintain iron, restoring haemoglobin to normal level. *Pregnant women should always seek the advice of a doctor before taking any medicines.*

Angina

Angina pectoris is caused by an inadequate supply of blood to the heart which impedes the blood flow through a narrowing of the arteries. It usually comes on suddenly, causing severe chest pains, often spreading to one or both arms and to the neck, throat, jawbone or back. Other symptoms (which usually occur after exertion or overexcitement) include nausea, feelings of suffocation or exhaustion.

The pains are very frightening, but angina does not usually cause permanent damage. The blood supply is never cut off, and there is no death of heart tissue, but the condition needs thorough medical investigation and treatment to ensure that the arteries do not continue to narrow.

A traditional Chinese doctor would expect patients to have had an ECG at an orthodox hospital to find out the extent of damage to the heart, and a number of Western drugs are very effective. To help prevent angina attacks, the patient could then take herbal medicines such as cinnamon twigs, safflower, red sage root, red peony root or macrostem onion bulb. Several herbs help to thin blood down, reduce cholesterol and triglyceride levels, which are contributory factors in atherosclerotic heart disease, and open the blockage.

Anorexia

This very complicated condition, often called the 'slimmer's disease', is usually suffered by teenage girls who develop a phobia against eating and a fixation about weight gain. The condition is connected with psychological problems which need to be investigated. Some doctors believe it may be triggered at puberty by an unconscious aversion to the changes taking place in their bodies, and a refusal to grow into maturity.

Sufferers also develop a weakness in their digestive system and the intestines and spleen must be strengthened. When the body has been without adequate food for a long time, the digestive system suffers in the same way as an unused muscle. Chinese medicine is often highly successful in restoring this function and helping the process of food digestion.

When the treatment takes effect, the bloated feelings which anorexics complain of after eating should be alleviated. Herbs prescribed to increase the appetite include rice sprouts, wheat sprouts and radish seeds or loganberry fruit. Although herbal remedies can, and do, restore health, it is a long process and constant support and psychotherapy are necessary.

Anxiety

Abnormal feelings of anxiety, as distinct from the natural reaction we all have to stressful situations in our daily lives, are an emotional problem which can produce physical symptoms ranging from panic attacks, nausea and vomiting to palpitations, hyperventilation and diarrhoea. Chinese doctors regard anxiety as the result of depression of the energy in the liver and a weakness of the spleen. The liver energy must be moved and the spleen strengthened using medicine which includes Chinese angelica and ginseng. Thorowax root used together with white peony root will also help relaxation.

Arthritis

Two of the commonest forms of arthritis are osteoarthritis and rheumatoid arthritis. Osteoarthritis usually affects the hips, knees, spine and hands, causing them to swell and stiffen. The condition is caused when the cartilage between the bones of the joints becomes worn, so that the bones rub against each other when the joints are flexed, causing intense pain.

Rheumatoid arthritis also involves swelling and stiffness and pain in the joints. It is characterized by feverish attacks during which the tissue, tendons and ligaments of the joints become inflamed and the skin swells and becomes very tender. Women are more prone to both forms of arthritis than men. The condition may be hereditary, and it may also stem from some form of allergy or be brought on by injury or stress on the joints.

In Chinese medicine the treatment of arthritis is divided into two major types. Herbal medicine is effective in reducing the swelling in acute arthritis, and acupuncture is usually good for helping to relieve the pain. Both kinds of arthritis are caused by 'wind damp', but one is the result of wind cold and the other of wind heat. In cold arthritis the joints are painful, particularly in the winter. Warming herbs will be used to clear the wind and dampness and to release the energy which has become congealed. These herbs include cinnamon twigs, pubescent angelica root or aconite root and wild ginger. When heat is the cause of arthritis, there is swelling and heat in the joints and corktree bark and large-leaved gentian are prescribed.

When patients seek treatment in the early stages of the condition, herbal medicines can be extremely effective. In more long-term cases, TCM can help to contain the arthritis, but if the joints are badly affected, their function cannot be restored.

Acupuncture can often give pain relief in severe cases, and is used in many Western hospitals.

Arteriosclerosis

Often called 'hardening of the arteries', arteriosclerosis is a factor in the ageing process when the arterial walls lose tone, and the circulation is affected. Symptoms include spells of dizziness, general weakness or blurred vision, and in severe cases there can be a risk of thrombosis or stroke. In TCM, the causes are very complicated. Two major contributory factors are the blood vessels and the blood itself. The heart, kidneys, spleen and liver are all involved in the quality of the blood. If it is too thick and has a high fat content, the blood vessels also thicken, sometimes causing the blood to move too slowly or to become stagnant.

To improve the circulation, Chinese angelica and soto ginseng, or perhaps red sage will be used. Then the quality of the blood must be upgraded, by strengthening and tonifying the spleen and kidney and balancing the liver. Hawthornberry, wolfberry, red sage and peach kernel, saffron, peony root, cinnamon and orange peel will help. If the problem is long-term or severe, a Western doctor should always be consulted.

Asthma

There are many causes of asthma – hereditary factors, an allergy to environmental influences such as dust or animal hair; or stress, anxiety or physical exertion. Western treatment includes the prescription of cortisone and inhalers that open up the bronchial passages. Childhood asthma often disappears after a few years, but it can develop at any time in adults, and although most attacks are of short duration, medical help should always be sought if the attack is serious and lasts for an hour or more, as the condition can be fatal.

In TCM, three organs are said to cause this problem: the lungs, the spleen and the kidneys. The major cause is phlegm produced by a weakness of spleen and kidney, but a Chinese doctor will identify the cause and nature of the complaint according to the patient's individual medical history.

Some cases respond well to kidney tonics, but if the problem is in the spleen, a different treatment will be tried. If it is the lungs which are deficient, the treatment will be geared to treating that organ. The intention is to open the lung energy to enable it to descend and clear the air passages. Herbs such as ephedra and bitter almond seed will help to stop wheezing. The Churchill Hospital in London has been conducting clinical studies into the effects of acupuncture on asthma, and hospitals in Oxford are researching herbal treatments. Asthma responds to both herbal medicine and acupuncture, although there have been recorded cases of acupuncture actually inducing an attack in susceptible patients, and it should of course only be administered in skilled hands (see case history, page 54).

Back pain
There are many causes of back pain and a doctor must first establish whether the problem is muscular, spinal, nervous in origin or caused by a disease of the internal organs. Back problems which are caused by strained or weak muscles or sciatica can be helped by herbs. Acupuncture, manipulation or massage may also be prescribed, and ointment, creams or plasters may be given. Chinese ginseng root, teasel root and acanthopanax bark are used to help relieve pain.

Bad breath
The spleen, which in TCM also involves the stomach, is the organ which dominates the mouth. If there is damp heat in the stomach, it can cause bad breath. The intestines are considered to be blocked. Medicines used to clear the problem and restore the breath to freshness include Chinese golden thread, giant hyssop and peppermint tea. Herbs such as radish seeds and oriental wormwood (a type of grass) may also be prescribed to help the digestion.

Baldness
Baldness is often due to hereditary factors and as such is difficult to treat. Where hair loss is caused by illness or chemotherapy, or where there is no history of baldness in the family, it can sometimes be helped by herbal medicine and acupuncture. The Chinese theory is that hair is nourished by the blood (which is dominated by the liver) and by the essence of the kidney. Liver and kidney deficiencies are considered the likely causes of baldness, so treatment will involve tonifying both organs. A good treatment is fleece-flower root. Wolfberry fruit or mulberry fruit can also help.

Bell's palsy
This is caused by damage to muscles on one side of the face due to swelling of the facial nerve. It very often occurs suddenly, sometimes overnight. It can be accompanied by pain in the affected side of the face, or in the ears. In TCM terminology, it is caused by a wind cold attack in the channel, which blocks the meridian so that the facial muscles cannot operate properly. Some people recover spontaneously, although this can take from a few weeks to a year.

Many studies have been done in China which show that acupuncture is very effective in treating Bell's palsy when it is used promptly. Complete recovery can take place in one or two weeks. Herbs which will expel the wind and cold from the body and stop headaches include wild angelica, sage and cinnamon twigs.

Blood pressure

High blood pressure is diagnosed as internal wind in Chinese medicine. The liver yin and blood will be treated, using herbs to calm the wind such as chrysanthemum flowers, peony root and astragalus. However, some people suffer complications which will require different treatment. Low blood pressure is a deficiency of the qi, the blood and the heart. Ginseng, Chinese angelica and tonic qi herbs are prescribed.

Both high and low blood pressure can be treated successfully by TCM. The herbs used are very helpful in controlling the blood pressure, so that Western medicines can be slowly reduced, under careful monitoring by a doctor. At the same time, the medicine should improve the general well-being, reducing the gan ho feelings of anger and irritability which the condition often causes.

Bright's disease

This is an inflammation of the tiny filtering units in the kidneys called glomeruli, causing red blood cells and proteins to leak into the urine. Symptoms are smoky or red urine passed in small amounts, puffy ankles, due to fluid retention, nausea and vomiting, abnormal sleepiness or drowsiness, and a general feeling of illness. It must be treated quickly, as if many of the filtering units are affected, high blood pressure or kidney failure can result.

A TCM doctor would see this as caused by weakness not just of the kidneys but also of the spleen, accompanied by damp or heat invasion of the body. Antibiotics will help, but TCM works toward strengthening the kidneys and spleen. A diet will be recommended, avoiding damp and hot food (see Chapter 8). Herbal treatments are very effective, and can improve urination and tonify the affected organs. Water plantain, bamboo leaves, liquorice, dogwood and mulberry fruit will all be used.

Bronchitis

Despite the severity of the Chinese winter, this illness does not have its own name in China, where it would merely be called coughing. The reason why it is known elsewhere in the world as the English Disease is that the British seem to suffer from it more than other nations. It can certainly be treated, usually with success. Different treatment will be applied according to whether the bronchitis is acute or chronic.

If acute, the condition is normally due to external reasons such as wind, cold or heat invasion. Chronic bronchitis, which is what most people suffer from in Britain, is attributed to internal problems: deficiency of the spleen or lungs, or internal phlegm. Where Western medicine waits for the attack to occur and then treats it, the aim of TCM is to prevent the onset of an attack.

Sufferers who dread winter because it will inevitably herald the onset of the disease should begin treatment in late summer or early autumn. In this way, they should have fewer or less serious attacks, which can sometimes be prevented entirely. A doctor examining a patient in the summer would assess the severity of the condition, even in the absence of the illness, by means of the tongue, the pulse and the breathing. He or she will then concentrate on improving lung energy, using herbs such as plantain seed, fritillary bulb or balloon flower root, honeysuckle flowers, skullcap root, lilyturf root, mulberry leaf or gardenia fruit.

Bladder problems

Incontinence among elderly people is a much more common problem than is generally realized because often victims feel too embarrassed to talk about it. Over the age of sixty-five, one woman in every twelve and one man in every seven suffers from incontinence. In TCM a weak bladder causing urination at frequent intervals and also a leaking bladder are due to the weakness of the kidney qi or the kidney yang. If the kidneys are weak, the quality of the urine is poor, and this irritates the bladder. Treatment will involve strengthening the kidneys with herbs which include eucommia bark, dogwood, or even walnut. Golden Lock Tea or Sextone is also effective. In some cases, acupuncture will help. Herbs and acupuncture are usually used in combination in these cases.

Bulimia

This condition is closely related to anorexia. Sufferers, who are usually young women in their late teens and early twenties, indulge in secret bouts of bingeing on all sorts of food, and then take large doses of laxatives and make themselves vomit, in order to stop themselves gaining weight.

TCM regards the problem as caused by a weakness in the spleen and stomach. The bingeing and vomiting cause further damage to the liver. Physically it is very important to strengthen the digestion so that when the patient does eat, she will not feel so uncomfortable, and will enjoy the food more. Tea made from hawthornberry, rice sprouts, wheat sprouts and even chicken gizzard are helpful. Chinese remedies like the Six Gentlemen can also help to strengthen the spleen and the stomach (see Chapter 12).

Cancer

Centuries ago, cancer was recognized in China as body tissue growing out of control, with potentially fatal results. It has a long history of treatment by traditional herbal medicine, as recorded in some of the ancient medical books. Researchers are studying cancer treatment with herbs in mainland China today. Every large university and teaching hospital is investigating old remedies, and the studies are producing promising results, usually in conjunction with Western treatment.

There are some ways in which Chinese medicine can help cancer cases where Western medicine cannot. Various herbal prescriptions have been shown to help in bolstering the immune system and some herbs can actually attack the abnormal cells and viruses which are responsible for certain types of cancer. Treatment aims first to increase the body's own defence mechanisms, then to kill the cancer cells.

Effective though radiotherapy and chemotherapy may be, they tend to have a drastic effect on the body generally, and patients often feel very tired and weak, and suffer from stress, anxiety and fear, and insomnia and loss of appetite. Chinese doctors regard strengthening the patient psychologically and physically to be of primary importance. Traditional herbal remedies can help reduce or eliminate the side-effects from radiotherapy or chemotherapy. Astragalus will help raise the blood cell count, the sickness caused by chemotherapy can be relieved with fresh ginger and orange peel, and acupuncture can also help. To attack the cancer itself, depending on type and location, different herbs will be used. A doctor will decide whether the illness is the result of qi energy deficiency, blood deficiency or yin or yang deficiency. Ginseng, astragalus, Chinese angelica, cooked rehmannia root, wolfberry root, Chinese yam and many tonic herbs may be used. But it is vital to remember that no one tonic is good for everybody. All treatments are dependent upon the individual. Some anti-cancer herbs used are usually very strong and sometimes make people sick, but this is because one poison is being used against another. How they work, and how clinically effective they are, is still being researched, and no claims can be made for them based on modern scientific evaluation.

Acupuncture and meditation are also very important parts of the Chinese traditional approach to the treatment of cancer. These alleviate pain and induce a sense of calmness, instil confidence and build up the spirit of the body, so that patients do not need to take so many painkillers. In China, they have many meditation programmes which are used to treat cancer.

Candida

Caused by dampness in the body. Sufferers should avoid sugar and dairy products. Treatment involves drying up the damp with pinellia tuber, poria, magnolia bark and kapok flower.

Cataracts

A relatively simple operation can restore the vision, but people who dislike the idea of surgery may find that TCM can enable them to live with the condition, if the sight is not too badly impaired by the time they seek help. It is diagnosed as a weakness of the liver and kidneys, due to lack of nourishment of the blood.

If patients consult a doctor at the outset, herbs can be prescribed which will slow the growth of the cataract and often stop it from developing any further, so that the sight will remain, if not perfect, then at least comfortable. The essence of the liver and kidneys and the blood will all be nourished by a treatment with rehmannia, wolfberry, chrysanthemum and dendrobium stem.

Catarrh

Nasal catarrh responds to peppermint, blackberry leaves and magnolia flowers. Patients will be advised to make changes in their diet and have extra seasoning in their food, including plenty of ginger and orange peel.

Chickenpox

This is a common children's disease caused by a combination of wind, damp and heat, which can also affect adults. It is highly infectious, but usually mild in childhood. Symptoms start with a raised temperature and an itchy rash covering the body, limbs, face and head. The spots are pink at first, then turn into blisters and then scabs. The virus remains infectious until the spots disappear after about five days.

Two forms of treatment are involved. Toxins must be eliminated from the body through the skin. The spots and blisters are encouraged to come out quickly. Many flowers such as saffron, honeysuckle and chrysanthemum will expel toxic substances from the body. Then the blood must be cooled by draining herbs, which will clear the urine and expel more toxins that way, to prevent the skin from scarring.

Chilblains

Caused by bad circulation, these are usually more of a female problem than male. Chilblains are characterized by a yang qi deficiency. Cinnamon twigs, red sage, dried ginger, aconite root can all be used to treat them. The best way to prevent chilblains is to wear warm clothing and take regular exercise to improve the blood circulation to the skin. Smokers should try to give up tobacco, as nicotine reduces the circulation.

Childbirth

Acupuncture will alleviate labour pains and can greatly assist any woman with a previous history of difficult labour. Any woman wishing to use this method of pain relief should consult an acupuncturist well before the birth date in order to build up a good patient-therapist relationship, but it is also necessary to obtain the approval of the midwife if it is a home birth, or the medical authorities if it is to take place in hospital.

There have been cases where hospitals were willing to allow an acupuncturist to assist at the birth, but only if they agreed to sign an indemnity form which absolved the hospital of responsibility if any problems ensued. Naturally, since complications not connected with acupuncture are equally possible at any point during a delivery, therapists are reluctant to shoulder such a burden. Any woman who wishes to have acupuncture during labour will probably find it easier to arrange if she gives birth at home, with a sympathetic midwife as supervisor. General debility following labour can be effectively treated by herbal remedies.

Chill

Anyone who feels the cold severely in winter will be treated with herbs to stop the cold atmosphere invading the body. Ginger will expel the cold, wind and damp from the body when boiled together with the white part of a spring onion, plus a little brown sugar for sweetness, and drunk as tea. This is a familiar home remedy in China.

Colic

Babies have an immature digestive system and also tend to swallow a lot of air with their food. Both contribute to colic. Gentle massage on the back, around the area of the spine, working from the bottom to the neck and pinching the spine very gently can help significantly. Do this every day, and it should alleviate the problem. If the problem is severe, consult a TCM doctor who will prescribe some herbs.

Colitis

Chronic inflammation of the colon is an extremely painful condition marked by frequent bouts of blood-streaked diarrhoea. If the patient has not already undergone food allergy tests, these should be undertaken before treatment begins. The condition has a variety of causes, from deficiency and cold in the stomach and spleen to dampness and heat, qi stasis, blood or food stagnation or possibly a yin deficiency. This is a troublesome and relatively common complaint which seems to respond rather more positively to TCM remedies than to modern medicine, which usually treats the patient with steroids or by surgery to remove the most severely affected parts of the colon. Dandelion, poria, astragalus, peony and ginseng may be used (see case history, page 54).

Conjunctivitis

Inflammation of the membrane which covers the white of the eye and the inside of the lids. It is often caused by a virus or by bacterial infections, but allergy or other factors can cause the problem. The eye becomes red and sore, and sometimes emits a sticky, yellowish discharge. TCM attributes the condition to wind heat, and it cases are mild, it can be treated without consulting a doctor. Sufferers should drink plenty of liquids, particularly herbal teas such as chrysanthemum or honeysuckle, both of which are very effective in expelling heat. Self-heal or bamboo leaves may be prescribed. The teas can also be used to wash the eyes externally. The washing should be done twice daily, when the water is just warm. If the condition is acute, or develops after a visit to a tropical country, it is wise to seek early medical advice, as the symptoms may indicate something more serious.

Constipation

Old people suffer from constipation when there is a kidney and spleen energy deficiency. A blood weakness can also be responsible, or a yin deficiency. Younger people suffer when there is a stagnation of stomach or liver qi, if they are stressed or anxious. Constipation can be a problem in pregnancy, when the foetus is causing internal pressure leading to a blood deficiency. Indigestion caused by overeating or eating the wrong foods can also contribute and in such cases a change of diet is advocated. Old people should be given sesame seeds, sprinkled on their food, or even sesame seed oil. This will also help in pregnancy.

In younger people who are not eating wisely, the system should be purged by rhubarb or magnolia bark used in combination. When the cause is stagnation of stomach or liver qi, the remedy called the 'Free and Easy Wanderer' (see page 130) is very useful. Plenty of greens will help, and spicy foods should be avoided. If these self-help methods do not cure the problem, consult a TCM doctor who will prescribe herbs to open the bowels, and will get to the root of the problem to discover why the bowels are not working.

Corneal ulcer

Often caused by a scratch on the cornea, the transparent covering which protects the lens of the eye. The white of the eye becomes bloodshot and waters, and there is pain and discomfort. A combination of allopathic and TCM therapy is the best recourse in these cases.

Antibiotics are very effective, but internally Chinese herbs can offer a lot of help to dispel the heat and fire in the liver and gallbladder. This will be cleared using skullcap and rhubarb, and will help to reduce scarring on the eyes. Herbal teas to wash the eyes can also help, in addition to antibiotics.

Crohn's disease

This is caused by inflammation of the ileum near the large intestine. It is recurrent, though there can be weeks, months or sometimes years between attacks. Symptoms include diarrhoea, and cramping pains after a meal, and the condition reduces the absorption of food, leading to a general feeling of debility.

Surgical operations are sometimes performed in severe cases, but are not always successful. TCM sees it as a condition caused by weakness of the kidneys and also sometimes of the spleen. Treatment will be aimed at helping the kidneys to improve the quality of the blood, so that the antibodies will increase in the bowel, allowing it to safeguard itself. Tonifying the kidneys is more important than treating the bowel alone. The stomach and spleen must also be treated, and a strict diet followed. This is not an easy problem to solve. Herbs used include aconite, poria, dried ginger and astragalus.

Deafness

Acupuncture is often used in China when deafness follows an infection, or even in some types of inherited deafness, though not always successfully. Mucus in the ears following an infection will be treated by herbs such as peppermint, thorowax root, plantain seed, chrysanthemum flowers, balloon flower root and Chinese gentian, self-heal and bitter almonds. In old people, in cases of deafness or tinnitus caused by age, the kidneys would be tonified using black ginger seed, dodder seed, mulberry fruit or eclipta and eucommia bark. This can be successful in reducing tinnitus and there should be an improvement in the hearing, or at least a halt to the deterioration.

Depression

The stress of everyday life makes this an increasingly common problem. There are two types of depression, the kind which stems from pressing problems or emotional upsets such as unemployment, debt, divorce or bereavement. This is called exogenous depression. The second type results from a chemical imbalance in the brain, and is known as endogenous depression. The first type can lead to the second, if help is not forthcoming, or if the exogenous depression does not improve through time.

TCM sees depression principally as a problem caused by liver qi stagnation. Normally the treatment would involve moving the qi and balancing the liver with herbs such as thorowax root, Chinese angelica root, white peony root and liquorice, or sometimes skullcap root. Free and Easy Wanderer is one of the best medicines for this. The holistic approach of TCM will involve the use of herbs to correct the chemical imbalance of the body, after which the depression will lift on its own. Physical and mental illnesses are inseparable to a Chinese herbal doctor.

Diabetes

The condition stems from the inability of the pancreas to produce enough insulin to regulate the blood sugar level in the body. Milder cases can be controlled by diet, but in many cases, daily injections of insulin are necessary. TCM can be very successful. It is generally considered a stomach, kidney and spleen problem.

Called 'sweet urine disease' in China, diabetes was recognized centuries ago and recorded in ancient medical texts, where it is described as 'three too much and one too little'. In other words, sufferers pass too much urine, are constantly thirsty, and therefore drink too frequently and often eat too much. Victims can also get very tired and thin.

There are well-documented cases of diabetics who were cured by herbal treatment, including those who were insulin-dependent. Sometimes it is also considered to be a lung problem caused by heat in the body through a yin deficiency. A doctor will clear heat from stomach, lungs and kidneys and will nourish the spleen, stomach and kidney. Lilyturf root, grassy privet, lotus seed, Chinese yam and mulberry fruit are used, as well as dogwood fruit and water plantain tuber. Diabetics who are insulin-dependent cannot be treated by a herbalist alone, but under the close supervision of a Western doctor they can then start taking herbs to improve their condition. Often this leads to a reduction in the amount of insulin they need, and it also helps the eyesight, heart and kidney functions which can be affected by the condition.

Diarrhoea

It should be stressed that anyone who experiences a persistent change in their normal bowel movement should always consult a doctor. If, however, there is nothing serious underlying the condition, it can be helped by herbal medicine. Dandelion, golden thread, skullcap root and kapok flowers would be used for acute diarrhoea. For chronic and persistent cases, astragalus, psoralea fruit and codonopsis root would be tried.

Dizziness

Chronic dizziness such as that caused by high blood pressure is considered to be the result either of liver heat or kidney deficiency. If it is acute, after infections like flu, it is regarded as an invasion of wind. This is expelled with herbs such as cinnamon twigs, peppermint, fresh ginger. Dizziness caused by internal problems may be treated by nourishing the blood with mulberry fruit, Chinese angelica and wolfberry, and a very effective fungus called gastrodia tuber is traditionally used.

Dysentery

The type of dysentery which affects people in Britain is a bacterial infection, caused by eating contaminated food or water, and spread by poor hygiene. Symptoms include severe blood-streaked diarrhoea, stomach pains, sickness and fever. Hygiene is extremely important as the condition is infectious. Amoebic dysentery is prevalent in tropical countries, and is a serious condition, requiring immediate medical attention. TCM regards dysentery as an external disease, considered to be due to heat and damp poison in the intestines, which causes a blockage. The medicine used for it includes treatment with anemone, which is very effective, plus white peony root, skullcap root and golden thread.

Eczema

There are many different types of this skin disease, which in TCM is associated with the lungs, stomach, heart and blood. One type is caused by damp heat, where the skin is weeping and there is a discharge with a sensation of heat and itchiness. Another cause is heat in the blood, where dryness, redness and itchiness are the symptoms, and the third kind, caused by wind, is an allergy where the skin erupts. Treatment is given accordingly.

Oriental wormwood or Chinese gentian, peony root and rehmannia are used for the eczema caused by wind. Schizonepeta and ledebouriella root are often chosen for other types. There are other more complicated forms. A Chinese doctor will diagnose these and treat accordingly. The condition usually responds well to TCM although it should be stressed that it does not work in every case.

Dermatologists working on a research programme at Great Ormond Street Hospital for Children have, in co-operation with TCM doctors, developed a more palatable teabag treatment. It is easier for the children to drink, but the results are not quite as impressive as those the Chinese doctor gets using pure TCM methods. They are, however, a big improvement over what was achieved in the past with Western medicine, and the future is very encouraging. A dermatologist from Tianjin hospital working at the Bath Medical Centre has also devised her own teabag granules which are easier to take and prepare than raw herbs. They are entirely based on TCM formulae.

Emphysema

This is a progressive and incurable disease which often affects very heavy smokers, or people who have worked with pollutants, or sometimes asthmatics and those who suffer from chronic bronchitis. It impairs the elasticity of the lungs, and therefore affects the circulation. This puts further strain on the heart which has to work harder to pump the blood, and can eventually lead to heart failure. TCM treatment will attempt to strengthen the lung along with the heart and kidneys. If the heart action can be strengthened, it can help the circulation and improve the blood supply to the lung. If the kidneys are made stronger it can help the lung to function more effectively and thus improve respiration. In Chinese medicine it is believed that the air breathed in by the lungs is 'grasped' by the kidneys. When the kidney is bolstered, the body fluids will improve, so that inside the lung there will be less mucus blocking the air passages. Remedies like the Six Gentlemen will help, but every case is different and the doctor will prescribe accordingly. Treatment is very difficult.

Enuresis (Bed-wetting)

After three years of age in children, this can be considered a problem. Most children have mastered day-time bladder control by that age, and the majority of them will also be dry at night. However, there is no need to worry if a child is sometimes slower. Children develop at their own pace. Making a fuss could put a strain on the child and may create a problem where none need exist.

Psychological problems can often lie at the root of bed-wetting which suddenly happens in older children. Upsets in the home or worries at school may be responsible, if there is no urinary infection or bladder problem. If it persists, consult a doctor.

TCM treatment will concentrate on the physical problems. One of the functions of kidney energy is to hold urine, and if it is weak the child will not be able to control its bladder. Herbs to tonify the kidneys and consolidate energy are walnut, chicken gizzard and black ginger seeds. These ingredients can be included in meals. Chicken gizzard, in dried form, can be bought at Chinese herb stores. In China, it is often sprinkled over the child's food.

Epilepsy

There are two common forms of this condition, which results from excessive electrical discharges in some of the nerve cells in the brain. Childhood epilepsy is called Petit Mal, and the fits, which are very brief, sometimes pass unnoticed. The child may sit rigidly staring ahead, while the eyes blink rapidly, and the hands and arms may jerk. He or she will lose consciousness only momentarily, and the attacks usually cease by the end of the teens.

Adult epilepsy involves attacks which can be very alarming, lasting for several minutes, in which the sufferer can froth at the mouth and thresh about. It is a common complaint, often hereditary, which affects about five people in every 1,000. People who suffer from epilepsy are forbidden by law to hold a driving licence, unless they have been free of attacks for two years. Severe and repeated attacks can result in permanent brain damage.

TCM regards epilepsy as a problem caused by phlegm blocking the orifice of the heart, plus internal dampness and qi or blood stagnation. Therefore the heart, spleen and even sometimes the liver will be treated. It is a very difficult condition to cure, and treatment is complicated, involving herbs such as sweet flag root, Chinese senegar root, bamboo shavings or bamboo juice from young shoots. If the patient does respond to treatment, herbal remedies can stop the fits in some cases, and cut down the number of attacks in others, as well as enabling the prescription of chemical drugs to be reduced, but it is a long-term treatment and not always successful (see case histories, page 57).

Exhaustion

When this is not simple tiredness such as would naturally follow a period of unduly hard or intensive work, physical or mental, it is considered a qi and blood deficiency: Korean ginseng is good for energy deficiency, other herbs include royal jelly and astragalus.

Eyesight

Poor eyesight is sometimes hereditary. Herbs which can improve vision are those which nourish the blood. These include wolfberry fruit, mulberry fruit, chrysanthemum flowers, cassia seed and fleece-flower root. Eyestrain is often caused by working in artificial light, or poor natural light, or for long hours in front of a visual display unit.

People who spend their working day in front of a VDU should ensure that they take a screen break every two hours for at least ten minutes. At home, reading or watching television, make sure that there is a good source of light, and relax the eyes from time to time by looking up from the page or the TV screen for a second or two every half hour.

Flatulence

Stagnation of the stomach energy, causing food stagnation and damp heat or indigestion. Normally doctors treat with magnolia bark, orange or citron peel. Another herb, amomum villosum fruit, called 'grains of paradise' in English, is often used, as is perilla stem.

Food poisoning

The commonest causes of food poisoning arise from poor hygiene or contaminated food. Reheating food, or not ensuring that it is cooked or stored properly, provides a perfect climate in which bacteria can flourish. There are various forms of food-poisoning germs. Salmonella and staphylococcus are two of the most familiar. Lysteria, which thrives in soft cheeses and pates, can pose a hazard for pregnant women, as it can affect an unborn baby. These items are best avoided in pregnancy. In food poisoning the lining of the stomach and the intestines become inflamed, causing vomiting, diarrhoea and abdominal pains. Fresh ginger or basil are frequently used in treatment.

Forgetfulness

This is usually age-related, and elderly people find it increasingly difficult to remember names or telephone numbers. Chinese medicine can be helpful. Poor memory is seen as a deficiency of the kidney essence. Treatment includes tonifying the kidneys with black ginger seeds, dogwood fruit, dodder seed and mulberry fruit. There will not be a quick result, but in the long term there will be an improvement. Acupuncture is also helpful in sharpening the memory.

Frozen shoulder

In China, this condition is called 'Fifties Shoulder' because it often affects people over that age, when their energy is declining through a weakening of yang qi. Water in the body can congeal into dampness which stagnates in the shoulder joint. This usually starts with inflammation of the tendons in the joint, or inflammation of the joint itself. There is a complex network of muscles and bone at the shoulder, because of the wide range of movements which the arms constantly have to perform. Movement becomes extremely painful, if not impossible, but it is important to try to keep the joint moving, otherwise the stiffness and pain will worsen and can result in permanent damage.

Acupuncture is the most effective treatment. Massage is also used, as is acupressure, and both can be effective. Herbs can be prescribed, the best being cinnamon twigs, which helps the energy to move to the hands and shoulder joints. Turmeric is also good.

Gallstones

It is quite possible to have gallstones without being aware of them. They are usually small pebbles formed from liquid bile, and the problems start when they get stuck in a duct, trapping bile in the gallbladder or blocking the flow of fluids from the pancreas. The symptoms include pain in the upper abdomen and tenderness under the ribs on the right side of the body, accompanied by nausea and vomiting.

TCM doctors say they are caused by damp heat in the liver and gallbladder. There are different types of gallstones. If they are very large, an operation is the best solution. Those which are less than 1.5 cm/ 1/2 inch in circumference can often be successfully dissolved or expelled by herbal medicine. The burning damp is believed to concentrate into stones, in much the same way as boiling sea water will produce salt. Herbs used in the treatment include lysimachia, pyrrosia leaf and rhubarb.

In China, large stones are sometimes treated internally, but the regime includes a stay in a TCM hospital where an intensive course of extremely strong herbal medicine is used to dissolve them, and so avoid the need for surgery. This is a common practice, successful in most cases, but it calls for constant observation by the doctor over a period of several days, and since there is not, as yet, a TCM hospital in Britain, it cannot be carried out here.

Gastric ulcer

Raw areas appear on the walls of the stomach where the protective mucus coating has worn away, possibly because of regurgitation of bile or over-production of acid. Food allergies, stress, certain drugs and poor eating habits, heavy drinking or smoking can cause the problem. Duodenal ulcers are much more common in men, and are caused by acid from the stomach forming raw patches on the lining of the duodenum, which results in a nagging pain in the upper abdomen a few hours after eating.

In TCM the treatment is the same for both gastric and duodenal ulcers, but there tends to be a higher success rate with duodenal cases. It is said to be caused by stomach qi and liver qi stagnation. The stomach and liver qi must be moved. Cyperus tuber, liquorice, dandelion, costus root or notoginseng root, ginger, skullcap root and magnolia bark will all help to achieve this. Treatments for both ulcer types are long term and involve dietary restrictions.

Genital herpes

This is caused by the Herpes Simplex virus and is very similar to the one which causes cold stores. The sores can be visible on the genitals and buttocks, but can also be found inside the vagina and anus. Itchy and painful blisters appear and leave ulcers when they burst. Glands in the groin become swollen and tender and sufferers often feel feverish and generally unwell. Symptoms usually clear within two weeks, but attacks frequently recur as the virus can lie dormant in nerve cells at the base of the spine. The condition is rare in China, but TCM doctors treating it in Britain consider it to be a problem of damp heat in the gallbladder channel. Chinese gentian, rhubarb, water plantain seed and plantain leaf are used in medicines.

Glandular fever

A viral infection spread by close personal contact, for example kissing. The disease incubates for as long as seven weeks, after which the patient develops swollen lymph glands on the neck, armpit and groin, enlarged tonsils with a white seepage, and often a much-enlarged spleen. There may be a rash similar to German measles, and jaundice may develop. The diagnosis is confirmed by a blood test, but there is no conventional treatment apart from painkillers to ease discomfort and reduce the temperature. Complete rest and plenty of liquids are important, and symptoms usually disappear by the second or third week, but the patient may take much longer to recover fully.

TCM views this as heat and phlegm in the blood, liver and stomach. The expanding heat causes the glands to swell and this must be cleared first. Red peony, dyer's woad leaf, honeysuckle, forsythia fruit, chrysanthemum flowers, dandelions, indigo and pigeon pea would be prescribed to clear the heat. The exhaustion which often accompanies the illness would then be treated with different herbal remedies.

Glaucoma

Caused by a build-up of fluid in the area between the cornea and the lens of the eye, due to blockage of the channel or the tissues through which fluid drains. This increases pressure on the eyeball, affecting tiny blood vessels at the back of the eye where nerve fibres from the retina enter the optic nerve, and leading to blurred vision. If the problem is acute, seek help from a Western eye specialist immediately, because the pressure can build up in the eye causing serious problems and possibly even blindness.

In TCM diagnosis, glaucoma is connected with the liver, gallbladder and stomach, and sometimes the kidneys also. It is identified with weakness in the liver and kidneys combined with heat and fire in the gallbladder and the liver. Fire ascending causes the eye problems, plus headaches and sickness. TCM will work internally, by helping to strengthen the kidneys and liver, reducing the fire and clearing the phlegm. Herbs and acupuncture will increase the speed of recovery and prevent recurrence. A famous remedy in Chinese medicine is called Dragon Bladder Purge Liver Decoction.

Glue ear

This is an accumulation of fluid behind the eardrum which is caused through blockage of the Eustachian tube. In TCM, it is caused by excessive dampness and heat in the body. It prevents the bones in the middle ear from vibrating properly, leading to increasing deafness. There may be a thick, smelly discharge, roaring or clicking noises in the ear, and swollen lymph glands. If not treated, the bones can become fused, leading to complete deafness. Allopathic treatment may involve minor surgery to remove some of the fluid, and inserting a grommet (a small tube) to allow the remainder to drain away. TCM treatment aims to eliminate damp and heat from the gallbladder channel. Avoid dairy products, sugar, spicy food and alcohol. Skullcap, rhubarb, plantain and peony will help. This is a complicated and long-lasting condition and hygiene is important. Sufferers must be careful when swimming, avoiding getting water in the ear. Herb drops can be put in the ear to clear the local infection.

Gout

Once believed to be the inevitable result of high living and over-indulgence in alcohol, gout is actually caused by an excess of uric acid and other compounds which accumulate in the blood. It can also be a painful side-effect of some modern medicines and diuretics. The intense pain and swelling in the joints is caused by acid and urate crystals and the crystals can also collect in the kidneys, causing kidney stones. Attacks often wear off after a few days, and may never recur, but repeated attacks can lead to permanent damage.

TCM doctors will treat patients for heat and damp in the blood and liver channel. Sometimes gout is also diagnosed as a kidney deficiency. The treatment is similar to that for kidney stones or arthritis. Herbs used in the medicine include bamboo leaves, Japanese thistle, akebia and flowering quince fruit. Acupuncture and moxibustion are usually effective in alleviating pain.

Guillian Barre syndrome

The peripheral nerves, outside the brain and the spinal chord, become inflamed in this disease, starting as tingling, numbness and weakness or paralysis affecting the hands and feet before spreading to the rest of the body. It is thought to be an allergic reaction to a viral illness or a vaccination, and the onset is very rapid. If the paralysis affects the breathing, intensive care in hospital is necessary. In two-thirds of the cases, a complete recovery is made in the first year or so, particularly in younger people, but it can be permanent. Acupuncture treatment may prove effective (see case history, page 66).

Haemorrhoids

Commonly called piles, haemorrhoids are caused by swollen or strangulated veins inside or on the exterior of the anus. They often protrude from the anus if the sufferer strains during a bowel motion, causing pain and bleeding. They sometimes stay permanently outside the rectum in the form of soft, grape-like purplish lumps. External piles usually clear up within a week or two, but sometimes leave small skin tags which cause further itchiness. Occasionally, blood inside a haemorrhoid clots, turning the pile into a hard and extremely painful lump.

All cases of anal bleeding should be medically investigated as they can indicate a more serious underlying condition. If the diagnosis shows the common problem of piles, which TCM sees as the result of heat, damp and blood stagnation in the anus, treatment will commence to move the stagnation, cool the heat and move the blood. Angelica, rhubarb, dandelion, magnolia bark and kapok flower are effective.

Hay fever

The balmy days of summer can be a complete misery for hay-fever sufferers, whose allergy to pollen released by grasses, flowers and trees means that they become unwell as soon as they put their head out of doors. The pollen causes cells to release histamine and other chemicals, resulting in blocked sinuses, a permanently runny, itchy nose, often a sore, irritated throat, watery eyes and constant sneezing. In very severe cases it can lead to asthma.

In TCM it is usually attributed to wind-heat invasion in the lungs. This is one of a set of atopic conditions that Chinese traditional medicine treats very simply and successfully. Eczema, hay fever and asthma are all conditions of atopy (a form of hypersensitivity, estimated to affect 10 per cent of the human race), so a treatment which works for one is quite likely to be successful in the other two.

Again, it must be emphasized that TCM treats each case individually, because symptoms vary between patients, and are also influenced by their particular experience and environment. In general, however, the doctor will open the lung qi to expel the wind heat. Herbs chosen for this could be magnolia flowers, chrysanthemum flowers, mulberry leaves, ephedra and cinnamon twigs (see case history, page 60).

Headache

Always consult your doctor if you develop sudden and recurrent headaches as they can be a factor in a variety of illnesses, some of which may be serious. However, for the everyday type of headache caused by tension, a simple Chinese remedy which you can make at home is spring onion tea. Use the white part of the plant only, and boil three or four onions in a mugful of water.

Headaches suffered after recovery from a stroke will be treated with lovage tuber. Wild ginger or wild angelica is used for migraine headaches. A Chinese doctor will suggest you seek hospital investigation without delay if a serious condition is suspected.

Migraine, in TCM, is connected with the liver, gallbladder and stomach, and caused by excessive stagnation of energy in the liver and gallbladder which then invades the stomach. The pain above the eyes, or flashing lights with pain in the forehead or sides ot the head, indicates involvement of the channels from the liver. The nausea which often accompanies migraine attacks is liver invasion of the stomach.

Treatment will concentrate on strengthening and tonifying the stomach, reducing the tension in the liver, moving the qi from the liver and gallbladder. Ginseng, poria, ginger, and Chinese date would be used for the stomach; skullcap, thorowax root and strong purging herbs such as Chinese gentian grass for the liver. Acupuncture is often effective in alleviating migraine attacks and Chinese meditation techniques can also help.

Heart disorders

Many very efficient drugs have been developed by Western medicine to alleviate heart conditions. Surgery is extremely sophisticated and routinely carried out to insert pacemakers or to by-pass affected arteries. In China, some of the most effective treatments have used a combination of both TCM and modern medicine.

A TCM doctor regards coronary heart disease as a yang qi deficiency, meaning that the force which moves the blood is weakened,- causing blood and qi stagnation which triggers the pain and the blockage. Treatment is started to warm the heart, tonify the energy, clear the blockage and move the blood. Palpitations are due to heart yin and blood deficiency and are caused by stress, fatigue, anxiety and nervousness.

The treatment aims to nourish the heart, lungs and blood. Many herbs effectively strengthen the heart energy and move the qi. Cinnamon twigs, aconite, dried ginger and red sage are good for moving the heart blood. In the TCM hospital in Tianjin, infusions of red sage and black aconite are given to heart attack victims and the recovery rate is much faster than with Western treatment alone. Herbs to nourish the yin and blood include lilyturf root, liquorice, dogwood fruit, wild jujube seed and Chinese angelica root. Modern pharmacological studies have shown that aconite has similar properties to the Western medicine digoxin.

Hepatitis

Hepatitis A is more acute, but easier to treat. It is a virus, affecting the liver, and spread through contaminated food or sewage. Symptoms resemble influenza at the onset, accompanied by nausea and loss of appetite. Jaundice follows and lasts for two to three weeks and the patient feels weak, depressed and generally run down for some months afterwards.

Hepatitis B is more serious. It has similar symptoms to the A virus, but can lead to acute liver failure or cirrhosis of the liver. The virus is transmitted by the blood or body fluids and some people are actually carriers without being aware of it until it shows up in a blood test.

No medical system can as yet claim an effective treatment for the B virus. As with cancer, there is promising research going on in China. Some herbs can improve the immune system. Treatment is always given on an individual basis. An acute attack causing jaundice is regarded as excessive damp heat from the liver and the gallbladder. Oriental wormwood is effective for this, and also gardenia fruit. Lack of energy, tiredness and pain associated with Hepatitis B would be treated with tonic herbs including

American ginseng, peony root, mulberry fruit, liquorice, dogwood fruit and grassy privet. Astragalus and Chinese angelica will strengthen the liver.

Hiatus hernia

Diet is important in this condition, which is due to a weakening of the tissue around the opening in the diaphragm. The stomach then protrudes up through the diaphragm, pressing on the valve between it and the oesophagus. Pressure prevents the valve from functioning properly, allowing acid from the stomach to well up into the oesophaghus, causing heartburn and sometimes pain in the neck and arms, which can be mistaken for angina. If the hernia is mild, no treatment is needed, but if it causes discomfort, acupuncture and herbal medicine can soothe the stomach and help digestion, relaxing the muscles. Magnolia bark, orange peel and ginger can help.

Hiccups

Even in a condition as seemingly simple as hiccups a Chinese doctor will look for a variety of causes. Hiccups can be the result ot heat, cold or food stagnation. Ginger, rhubarb and perilla stems are commonly used. Acupuncture can help in persistent cases, and during a short attack, a few minutes of acupressure applied to points at the top of the eye socket can often bring them to a halt.

Hodgkin's disease

A combination of TCM and Western medicine is often successful in treating this form of cancer of the lymph glands. It is one of the cancers which, in modern medicine, is curable in 90 per cent of cases. If chemotherapy and radiotherapy are used, TCM can alleviate the side-effects and bolster the body's ability to resist the disease. A TCM doctor would say it is caused because the kidneys, liver and spleen are not working well together. The kidneys and spleen must be strengthened, the damp heat and phlegm must be cleared from the body, and the blood must be moved. Acupuncture and whole body treatment are needed. The herbs used are very similar to those used in other forms of cancer.

Immune system

The Chinese use the term 'defence system', which is very similar. They consider it to be part of the qi. One of the undoubted strengths of TCM is its ability to influence the immune system, and clinical trials are going on all over China and elsewhere in the world to further medical knowledge about this. Infectious diseases and even epidemics have been controlled by acupuncture for centuries. Its use is much wider in China than here in the West. Research carried out at Beijing Children's Hospital showed that acupuncture was very effective in treating childhood dysentery. Certain herbs have been identified as acting on the immune system both as a booster (astragalus, wolfberry, ginseng) or suppressor (thorowax root, black plum).

Impetigo

A highly contagious skin infection, common among children, which often causes minor outbreaks in schools and kindergartens. The spots, red with a yellow crust, usually affect the face, hands and legs, but can spread over the rest of the body. The sores may last for weeks.

Although impetigo is an external condition, in TCM theory the real cause is toxins caused by heat and damp in the body, especially in a weak liver and kidneys. Treatment can be external and internal. If the condition is mild, herbs to wash the skin will be prescribed, or a herbal cream will be supplied. If the problem is severe, Chinese golden thread, gardenia fruit, skullcap or the bark of the mulberry tree will be used.

Hygiene is very important, and medical treatment should be started immediately because impetigo is highly infectious. Keep the skin and hands well washed and scrupulously clean. Other people in the family, or other children who come into contact with the disease, can use tea made from corktree bark to wash their hands, as it sterilizes the skin and stops the infection from spreading.

Impotence

The process of sexual arousal is such a complex and delicate operation in men, and so fundamental to their self-image, that it is not surprising so many things can go wrong.

An erection results when blood pumps into the spongy tissues of the penis, causing them to swell and stiffen. Hormonal activity, a response in the central nervous system, the emotions and the thought processes are all involved. With so many physical, psychological, neurological and chemical factors triggering a response, problems can easily arise. Often it is a temporary phase, following illness, stress or overwork, but many other subtle psychological factors may be involved. Occasionally, too, impotence can be a side-effect of drug therapy.

TCM has several preparations which can treat the problem. In young people, it is considered to be a weakness of the kidneys and the liver. Too much anxiety and stress can bring about liver qi stagnation, which weakens the kidneys and can occasionally cause impotence. No single treatment will help all cases, since the causes vary considerably, but in general a prescription called Sextone, and also cibot root and seahorse, can help.

Incontinence

In adults, the common problem of bladder incontinence often affects women after childbirth, and in men it may result from prostate problems. The treatment is similar to that used for bedwetting in children. It is often a kidney yang deficiency plus internal coldness. When the kidney energy is weakened, its function in holding water is affected in the same way as weakness in the human body makes it difficult for a sick person to close a heavy door. A familiar, usually effective remedy, is Golden Lock Tea.

Indigestion

Snatched meals, eating too quickly or overeating can lead to indigestion. Smoking, eating rich, fatty foods and drinking too much alcohol or coffee can also be contributory factors. The TCM view is that indigestion is normally due to a weakness of the stomach and spleen. Tonic herbs will be used to ease digestion and some kind of diet prescribed to control the appetite. Herbs such as hawthornberry, wheat and rice sprouts and chicken gizzard can ease the discomfort.

Infertility

The infertility file in the TCM doctor's London clinic makes very moving reading. There, among letters from desperate women asking if Chinese medicine can help them to conceive, are colourful birth announcement cards, photographs of newborn babies and in one note a request that the doctor suggests a Chinese name for a tiny boy, to celebrate the successful outcome of infertility treatment through herbal medicine.

A growing number of couples in Britain have had TCM treatment when all else failed, and found it worked for them. In mainland China, many research papers have been published about the techniques. TCM doctors have prescribed herbal medicine and given acupuncture to increase fertility in women and the male sperm count. Results have been encouraging.

Despite the fact that modem medicine can perform near-miracles for the childless, infertility remains a very common problem in Britain, affecting as many as one in six women, and about the same number of men. The causes are either functional, in which case there is nothing wrong with the reproductive organs yet the couple fail to conceive; or there is an organic reason, perhaps blocked tubes or an obstruction, or problems with the uterus.

In vitro fertilization (IVF) can overcome some of the organic difficulties, but still has a limited success rate (about 15 per cent). Sadly, long waiting lists and cost put IVF beyond the reach of many couples. For those who have no physical barriers, the mystery of why they fail to conceive often makes the problem worse. When you know something is wrong, you can look for a cure. When investigations show that everything is normal, and yet no baby arrives, the only advice is to go on trying. 'Hope deferred maketh the heart sick,' says the Bible, and only the childless know the anguish of waiting every month for a hope which seems to be endlessly deferred.

The Chinese answer to this is to seek the imbalance in the body itself. In TCM, there is *always* a reason one part of the system does not function as it should, and that reason may well lie somewhere else. Find out where it is, and the question is already half answered. Where fertility is the problem, the answer is very probably in the kidneys.

Life in the Western world brings its own fertility problems, according to TCM doctors. We drink too much coffee, drink too much alcohol, and eat too many sweet things which give false energy without any actual nourishment, giving rise to damp in the body, which causes blockages. Add to that an affluent lifestyle, when between the teens and thirties it is customary to have late nights and, in many cases, an active sex life, and you have all the factors which make a traditional doctor shake his head.

The Chinese have a different attitude to sex. It is part of the jing, the essential essence of life stored in the kidneys, and finite in quality. Too much sex can deplete the reserves of jing, so that later in life, when people settle down and start to think of having a family, the pool is low, making conception difficult. When stress comes into the picture, matters get worse.

The *Nei Jing*, the *Yellow Emperor's Classic of Internal Medicine*, the oldest and most revered Chinese medical classic, sets out the course of physical development and the wise way to sustain it. On the development of girls it states: 'At seven her teeth and hair grow longer; at fourteen she begins to menstruate and can bear children, at twenty-one she is fully grown and her physical condition is at its best.'

Of boys: 'At the age of eight his hair grows long and he changes his teeth; at sixteen he begins to secrete semen, at twenty-four his testicles are fully developed and he has reached his full height.'

In other words, the ideal ages for the beginning of a sex life, and procreation, are twenty-one for women and twenty-four for men. Doctors practising traditional medicine today believe that the wisdom of the ages is more relevant than ever in modern-day life. If people reserve the energy of the kidneys until the time when they want children, in a healthy couple, there will be no problem.

But when people start a sex life in their teens, combined with the high living of the materialistic Western world, they are damaging their own vital energy and endangering their chance of parenthood. This is particularly true when a young girl is put on contraceptives at an early age for menstrual problems, or to avoid pregnancy. According to the TCM view, if she stops taking the pill at thirty, and at last allows her ovaries to do their work, she has eighteen-year-old ovaries in a thirty-year-old body. This is a serious imbalance, and all disease stems from imbalance in the TCM view.

The ovaries may need to be treated to strengthen and support them. Other gynaecological procedures, such as D & Cs and abortion, may have caused scarring to the uterus. Anyone can see the effect of a permanent scar on the surface of the skin. It is a different colour, and a different texture, with a smoothness on the healed tissue. If there is scarring inside the small, pear-shaped uterus, then the surface will also have that slippery texture, making it difficult for the sperm to gain hold. Dampness in the uterus, sometimes the result of too much sugar in the diet, can also make it difficult to penetrate. Ask a TCM doctor why this should be so, and he will tell you to think of how quickly sugar goes damp and sticky in a bowl. The same thing happens in the body, he explains.

In treating women, the doctor's first concern will be to regulate the periods. Once the herbal treatment gets the blood moving, there should be normal blood loss and duration, neither heavy nor scanty, and the blood itself will begin to look fresh, not dark and clotted. Once menstrual regularity is achieved, the hormone balance in the body will improve automatically. The herbs will also alleviate pre-menstrual tension, which is often a factor in infertility. If those problems are solved, the woman's general energy and sexual libido will improve, and the kidneys will begin performing their hormonal functions efficiently. The ovaries will be working better, and the reproductive system will be producing eggs.

Treatment will also involve tonifying the spleen and nourishing the body generally. A dysfunction of the spleen produces dampness, affecting the lining of the womb and the heaviness of the bleed. The mucus caused by the dampness will be cleared away and eliminated throughout the system. The liver, too, has to be improved. It is responsible for the balance of the body, and if there is a blockage, the pain and PMT which this causes stems from the liver.

Many women who undergo fertility tests are found to have a blockage of the fallopian tube. Obviously, where the problem is as the result of surgery or a past infection, treatment will be more difficult or perhaps impossible. But where there is no definable cause, TCM doctors say this is exactly the same as blocked sinuses, and these can be successfully cleared in about half the cases. The treatment can also increase the chances of a successful outcome of IVF, because, in another of the metaphors TCM is so fond of, when the soil is well prepared beforehand, the harvest will be better.

In men, problems caused by underdeveloped or undescended testicles are difficult to treat, though not impossible. If the problem is functional, the major cause will be attributed to the kidneys. There may be a genetic weakness, or a history of too much sex too early in life. Smoking and alcohol have an adverse effect on the body, and fatty foods are also harmful. Deep-fried food dries the essence. Past illness and drug therapy, especially steroids, can have a detrimental effect on male potency and the patient will be advised to change his lifestyle.

Treatment in men concentrates on the kidneys, and if they respond, the amount, mobility and activity of the sperm will improve. Sperm production, in ordinary circumstances, can vary dramatically between one test and another. A reading taken one month may be 20 million, in another it may be 40 million in the same man. Temperature, environment and all manner of complex factors, general health high among them, can affect amount and quality.

But where a reading goes from 2 million in the initial test to 54 million after six months of TCM treatment, as it did in the case of a patient tested in St Mary's Hospital, Manchester in 1992, it seems not unreasonable to suppose that herbal medicine has had some influence on the improvement. Sperm tests in the case of Stephen K. showed that not only had the amount improved out of all proportion, but the quality of the sperm produced was equally marked. Mobility and activity gave readings of 80 and 90 per cent. Previously mobility was zero.

There is no conclusion to this story yet, as the patient's wife suffers from endometriosis and other menstrual problems. However, endometriosis is another condition which has a good record of response to herbal medicine, and Mrs K. has now started treatment with the same doctor. The couple are planning another IVF attempt in six months' time, and report that since receiving herbal medicine they both feel that their general health has improved markedly.

'The hospital originally told us that our chances of a baby were zero. We had a very understanding GP, who gave us every backing, and we got marvellous support from a private surgeon who told us that he could do nothing to help, but that there might be an answer out there somewhere, in some form of unconventional medicine, and that we should keep on looking for it,' said Stephen.

'We did so, and that was what led us to try TCM. My wife has an inverted uterus and several other menstrual problems, but now she has a normal cycle and she has never felt better. The TCM doctor told me I was in very poor physical shape, and it wasn't until I started taking his pills that I realized how true that was. Even if we never have a child, the treatment has been worthwhile.'

No genuine TCM practitioner would wish to give false hope to patients who have already despaired of finding a treatment to enable them to have a child. There are several barriers to conception for which only surgery or sophisticated laboratory techniques can provide the answer. The strength of well-known Chinese herbal treatments lies in helping the cases that are not organic in origin, where there is no identifiable cause of infertility, and when that is the diagnosis, any good TCM doctor should be able to help.

The approach obviously varies with the condition. One woman doctor practising in London is carrying out the techniques she used at the TCM Teaching Hospital at Canton, injecting herbal medicine direct into two acupoints. She, too, has a picture on file of a baby, born to a woman patient with a familiar case history of conception difficulties and failed IVF treatment. She conceived after eighteen treatments of herbal acupuncture, given on a twice-weekly basis.

There was a successful outcome for another couple after three years of Western infertility treatment elsewhere. Shirley was put on the pill at nineteen and took it for nine years before having an ectopic pregnancy, which meant that a fallopian tube had to be removed. She had bad period pains and PMT, and the coating of her tongue was peeling off at the root when a TCM doctor examined her, a strong indication of kidney weakness. At thirty-five, two previous IVF attempts had failed.

Her forty-year-old husband had a low sperm count with no activity. He was generally run down, and his kidneys were tonified with tonic herbs such as eucommia bark, mulberry, dodder seeds and ginseng. He was also given antelope horn to strengthen the essence of the kidneys. After six months of treatment the count was four times higher, and a third IVF treatment was tried. The couple now have a baby.

Fertility was not the problem for a thirty-two-year-old woman who sought treatment. Four pregnancies ended in miscarriage with the babies dying in the uterus between fourteen and sixteen weeks. The TCM doctor thought she might not be supplying enough blood for the foetus. He diagnosed a weakness in her general health and in her kidneys, and also prescribed to tonify the blood.

The patient had suffered from migraine, which is a weakness of the spleen, and therefore three organs were involved in the treatment, including the liver to nourish the blood. Her husband was also treated in case the sperm was weak. When she became pregnant, nine months afterwards, the doctor continued to monitor her condition, prescribing strong herbs from the tenth to the twentieth week. She gave birth to a healthy baby.

Even the TCM doctor was surprised at the outcome for one couple, who had tried seven IVF treatments without success. They already had an eight-year-old child, and the hospital could find no reason why the mother could not have another baby. In fact, she was in poor health with scanty periods, feeling tired and weak all the time. Four months after starting on a course of herbal medicine, she became pregnant.

The main problem stemmed from the male in a second case where a couple had a child but failed to have a second. The husband had frequent swollen glands and bouts of tonsillitis, he suffered from back pain and had been treated for non-specific urethritis (infection of the urethra often due to chlamydia, which is a cross between a bacterial infection and a virus). Urinary problems, back pain and throat complaints are all allied to the kidneys, the main organ of reproduction in TCM, so the doctor treated the kidneys with extra herbs to remove dampness from his body.

All TCM treatment is holistic and very much based on the individual symptoms and history of the patient. Not all cases will have a happy ending, and treatment often takes up to a year or more, regardless of the outcome. But the treatment is gentle and noninvasive, and will usually improve general health and alleviate or remove any menstrual disorders.

Influenza

A high fever with cold sensations, aching joints, sweating, headaches and general weakness, a cough and chest pain: most strains of the all-too-familiar flu virus have these symptoms in common. Western medicine advises bedrest, plenty of fluids and regular doses of aspirin or paracetamol as the best treatment. No modern medicines are effective against a virus, and this one changes its structure from year to year.

However, TCM offers a much more optimistic outlook. Flu is treated in three categories: wind cold, wind heat or damp, and treatment will differ slightly according to the type.

A large number of flowers and aromatic herbs will be used by a TCM doctor when treating this common complaint. Moxibustion is an effective therapy because a pungent aroma, which is made to rise through burning, can clear the toxins from the body.

In China, there are several well-known brands of patent medicines which are effective in treating flu and feverish colds. These are now proving popular over here, and are available from Chinese herbal shops on consultation with the pharmacist, who will advise on the one most suitable for the particular symptoms. Honeysuckle, forsythia, chrysanthemum, peppermint and cinnamon are among the herbs used.

Insomnia

This is a common symptom in a variety of mental illnesses, and in China, patients are often described as suffering from insomnia or restlessness when, in the West, the condition might be diagnosed as chronic depression or schizophrenia. Insomnia is considered to be connected with the heart, kidneys, liver and stomach, but particularly with the heart, which houses the shen, or spirit. The TCM view is that the spirit cannot rest, either because there is heat in the heart, or as a result of weakness in the kidneys caused by fire and water being out of balance. The heart is the organ of fire, while the kidney is the water organ. Water normally subdues fire, but if the kidneys are weak there is not enough water to do this and the fire can get out of control.

Overeating, or indigestion caused by a weak stomach, can also lead to insomnia. In TCM patients will never be given tranquillizers or sleeping pills. Instead, the doctor will try to find out the particular cause. Herbs regularly used are fleece-flower stem, poria, wild jujube seed. The herbs do not sedate the patient, but appear to have a beneficial effect on the nervous system. Sleeping on a gypsum pillow is a familiar Chinese do-it-yourself remedy for mild cases, and there is an effective do-it-yourself acupressure, massage and exercise routine which a doctor can demonstrate to patients. Acupuncture is widely and often very effectively used in the treatment of insomnia caused by depression and related emotional problems.

Irritable bowel syndrome (Spastic colon)

This is due to a weakness of the muscle action in the walls of the gut, which push down through the intestines into the colon and rectum. It causes spasmodic pain with explosive, watery diarrhoea, alternating with bouts of constipation. There is no physical cause for IBS, as it is usually called, but there are possibly psychological reasons, and a poor diet with insufficient fibre may also be to blame.

TCM regards it as an imbalance between stomach, spleen and intestines, sometimes also affecting the liver and kidneys. Normally it is a weakness of the spleen and kidneys, with too much dampness in the intestines, plus liver qi stagnation. It is not always an easy condition to cure, but the aim will be to tonify the spleen, clear the toxins from the body and balance the immune system. Dandelion is good for this purpose, while magnolia bark can ease the bloated feeling in the stomach, and rhubarb and Chinese angelica will stop constipation. Poria will control diarrhoea.

Itching

This may be caused by external wind, hot or cold, or sometimes internal wind. Dittany bark, puncture vine fruit and broom-cypress fruit are used for itchiness. In mainland China, doctors also use snake skin, because a snake is a cooling and cold animal, and therefore good for people who suffer from acute itchiness.

Snake skin, like many of the other ingredients in the traditional Chinese pharmacopoeia, is not a remedy which would be used in this country, though it has a number of applications in the Far East, including treatment for arthritis (a snake lives in water and damp ground and does not suffer from its lifelong exposure to that environment, so the theory goes that there must be components in its body which protect it).

Many of the more bizarre ingredients used in Chinese medicines are banned from import in this country, and thankfully, due to pressure from the international community, some of them are at last being prohibited from use in mainland China. Rhinoceros horn and tiger bone have now been banned there. TCM doctors here have hundreds of herbs at their disposal which are usually far more effective substitutes.

Jaundice

Characterized by a sickly yellow tinge to the skin and the whites of the eyes. The yellow pigment is called bilirubin, and is produced in the spleen when old or damaged red blood cells are destroyed. Normally the liver removes the bilirubin from the blood and sends it through the gallbladder and the bile duct into the intestines, where it colours the faeces brown. In someone with jaundice, the faeces are grey and chalky, and the urine is darker.

Jaundice can be a symptom of something more serious such as cancer or cirrhosis. It may also be caused by gallstones, or steroids and other chemical drugs. A blood test should be carried out.

In TCM it is a condition mainly connected with dampness in the liver and gallbladder. Herbs to clear the damp heat are very successful, particularly oriental wormwood and gardenia fruit. Corktree bark is also used. Jaundice due to liver cancer is considered to be a problem of blood stagnation, and herbs to clear the blockage would be used.

Laryngitis

Acute laryngitis is the result of an infection and causes pain and discomfort in the throat. A second type is chronic, much longer-lasting and recurrent. It can be caused by emotional stress or by aggravating the vocal cords through singing or straining the voice, also by smoke, fumes or dust. A bacterial infection which would be treated with antibiotics in orthodox medicine, laryngitis is regarded as heat and poison in the lung by TCM doctors. Acute cases would be treated with honeysuckle flowers, peppermint, liquorice, mulberry leaf and blackberry lily.

Leukaemia

Cancer of the blood cells. Many patients can now be cured. Major advances have been made in the treatment of the most common childhood leukaemia called acute lymphoblastic leukaemia. In adults, lymphoblastic and myeloid leukaemia can be either acute or chronic. Symptoms include fever, anaemia, headaches and excessive nose-bleeds, loss of energy and loss of appetite, weakness and weight loss. In women, it can result in extremely heavy blood loss at menstruation.

Chemotherapy and other orthodox medicine are all regarded as helpful by Chinese doctors but there are also some herbs which are quite effective and are being researched in China. Wolfberry, ginseng, astragalus and Chinese yam appear to be able to increase normal red and white cell counts, and to suppress the cancer cells.

Lichen planus

This is an intensely irritating skin complaint, which often causes flat papules on the limbs and body, and in extreme cases even on the membrane inside the mouth. In TCM terms, it is diagnosed as poisonous heat and blood stagnation. It can be caused by stress. Like many other skin conditions, it responds well to herbal treatment, and in fact there are some thirty-seven different herbal recipes well known to doctors, all in common use, and prescribed according to the nature and severity of the problem.

Ligament sprain

Chinese cupping and acupuncture, massage and herbal plasters are helpful, and the injury would be regarded as a problem of internal blood and qi stagnation. Herbal medicine would be prescribed to help move the blood and the qi using safflower, millettia stem and Chinese notoginseng root. The upper limbs would be treated differently from the lower limbs and the herbs chosen in order to act on the organ which is considered to be the cause of the problem.

Lumbago

Pain in the small of the back, sometimes brought on by lifting or when muscles are strained or torn and go into spasm. In severe cases, the back can seize up, leaving the patient unable to straighten up. A slipped disc or the displacement of vertibrae can also be responsible. X-rays or blood tests may be called for to establish the source of the trouble. If it is a straightforward case, acupuncture is generally very effective, particularly for acute conditions. If there is spinal trouble, some kind of manipulation may be necessary. Chronic lumbago, particularly in old people, responds well to TCM treatment. A tincture, or herbs which can be soaked in wine or spirits during the winter, will be prescribed to warm the body, improve the circulation and stop the pain.

Cibot rhizome, achyranthes root or acanthopanax bark can be put in alcohol or spirits. For problems caused by injury, a different treatment would be given. Acupressure and massage are also effective in treating many back problems.

Lupus

Lupus vulgaris, which usually attacks young people, affects the skin on the face and neck. *Lupus erythematosus* occurs in two forms, both more common in women. One form involves slightly raised red patches on the face, giving a characteristic butterfly appearance; the other can affect the internal organs. Both respond well to TCM. Herbs can control the disease and enable patients to cut back on the steroids they are prescribed in Western medicine.

Malaria

Common in southern China and South East Asia, malaria is spread by mosquito bites, which inject tiny single-cell parasites into the bloodstream. By this route, the parasites find their way to the liver, where they begin to reproduce, and then return to the bloodstream again, between nine and thirty days after the original bite.

The symptoms include headache, nausea and fatigue, and the sufferer begins to feel cold and shivery, followed by high fever, profuse sweating and a fall in temperature. Afterwards, the patient is left feeling extremely weak, and unless treatment begins immediately, further attacks are likely within days. Anyone returning from a visit to a known malarial region, and suffering from these symptoms, should seek medical help immediately, even if they have been taking anti-malarial drugs.

Conventional drugs like quinine are used in the treatment of malaria, but sweet wormwood is a famous herbal medicine. The Chinese herb qinghaosu, or artemisia, has been the subject of a study funded by the World Health Organization. It has long been recognized in China for its medicinal properties and is documented in ancient texts such as the *Materia Medica* of the Da-guan period of AD 1092.

Mastitis

Nodular mastitis is relatively common before a period is due. It is a harmless condition, but uncomfortable and often worrying. The lumpy, tender feeling in the breasts is caused by hormonal activity.

TCM treatment can be helpful in particularly troublesome cases. Mastitis is seen as the result of stagnation of the qi and the blood. The blood must be moved and the heat and poison expelled from the body. Madder root, burred tuber or costas root, peony bark, dandelion, snake gourd seed or Chinese gentian are normally used. A homemade concoction applied externally will ease the discomfort and hasten healing. This is made with powdered dried rhubarb root (which can be bought from a Chinese herbal store) mixed with olive oil.

ME (Myalgic encephalomyelitis)

The daunting name of this mystery illness actually means inflammation of the brain and the spinal cord, with associated muscular pain, but this is misleading. Another, more accurate name is postviral fatigue syndrome. The disease attacks every part of the body, leaving the patient extremely exhausted, entirely drained of strength, and often suffering from headaches, muscle pains, visual disturbances, sweating or shivering fits, frequently accompanied by loss of memory, lack of concentration, mood swings and depression. ME usually starts after a virus infection such as influenza or glandular fever. The virus which causes glandular fever has been found in some ME sufferers, but in others there are changes in the immune system and in the composition of the muscle cells. Stress may be another factor.

In TCM the exhaustion is considered to be a weakness of qi and a blood deficiency, as well as a damp heat problem. The doctor would tonify the energy and try to clear the damp. This condition exemplifies the differences between medical systems. While the debate about ME continues among some Western practitioners, a TCM doctor will check the pulses and the tongue, diagnose the syndrome and decide to which pattern of disease that particular case conforms.

In general, treatment will be aimed at helping the immune system to fight back, and a course including both acupuncture and herbal medicines is likely to be recommended. Recovery can take from three to six months in the case of young sufferers, but it is likely to be slower and longer-term in older patients (see case history, page 62).

Measles

A common childhood ailment which starts with fever, a dry cough and sore eyes, after which a brownish-pink rash breaks out over the whole of the body. There may also be white spots on the insides of the cheeks a day or two before the skin rash appears. The condition is usually mild in children (although it is still a major cause of death among children in the Third World) but in adults it can cause complications and recovery may take up to four weeks.

Measles in TCM diagnosis is caused by heat in the stomach and blood. The spots will be encouraged to come out quickly to detoxify the body. Crocus sativae and duck meat, peppermint and honeysuckle flowers are mainly used to bring the measles to the surface, with other herbs to detoxify.

Memory loss

When this problem is caused by serious brain damage, nothing can be done, but if it is the result of age, stress or tiredness after illness, it can be treated with acupuncture and herbs. The medicine would tonify the kidneys and strengthen qi and blood, as well as opening the channels to release nourishment to the brain. Chinese wolfberry, Chinese fleece-flower root and black ginger seeds can be used. Acupuncture is quite important in this treatment and there are special tiny needles for tonifying the kidneys and nourishing the brain. These are placed in the head and ears and can be taped on and left in place for days, without the wearer being aware of them.

Menière's disease

The result of too much fluid in the labyrinth of the ear. It may cause dizziness, lack of balance, nausea and vomiting, and may affect the hearing. TCM attributes it to a kidney weakness, as the kidneys are paired with the ear.

One of the other functions of the kidneys is to nourish the marrow which feeds the brain. If the kidneys are weak, the brain is improperly nourished, and dizziness and loss of balance are the result.

Another outcome of kidney weakness is internal cold. Therefore the water the kidneys normally process becomes mucus (phlegm) and a weakness develops in the spleen. This excess fluid goes into the ears, and treatment is needed to warm and tonify the kidneys and strengthen the spleen to clear away the gunge. Herbs will include the well-known Return Spleen decoction, Sextone, or Central Qi Pills. Astragalus, ginseng, orange peel, ginger or cinnamon bark are used. People with Meniere's disease should avoid 'cold' food such as salads, cold drinks or ice cream and also sugar and dairy products which can increase the dampness in the body and make more fluid, with which leading to further attacks. *Gastrodia elata* is a very effective herb to treat dizziness. A tang, a herbal soup, made with these ingredients, and drunk from time to time can help to prevent future attacks (see Chapter 8).

Meningitis

A viral or bacterial infection of the delicate membranes surrounding the brain. It can also be caused by a head injury. Symptoms are fever, nausea and vomiting with a stiff neck, and a severe headache, and an intolerance to light. Patients may become delirious, abnormally sleepy or drowsy, and can go into coma.

Viral meningitis is less severe and recovery usually comes within two to three weeks. The bacterial type can be more serious, and can result in deafness or brain damage, or even sometimes prove fatal. Meningitis in babies is potentially more serious than in older children and there is a risk of brain damage if the disease is not diagnosed and treated in the early stages. It begins with a high fever, with the neck held rigid or the back arched, and either unusual irritability or quietness, and turning away from light. There may be vomiting or convulsions plus an unusual high-pitched cry and a purplish rash on the trunk.

In infants, the fontanelle (the soft area on the top of the head where the skull bones have not yet knit) may bulge. This is caused by pressure of fluid around the brain. If meningitis is suspected, seek medical help immediately. The chances of a good recovery are high.

Herbal treatment for meningitis has been very successful in China. In the recent past there were many epidemics, particularly in the north, and the hospitals routinely used herbs as treatment, with a high degree of success. One famous remedy is called White Tiger Decoction, the main ingredients of which are gypsum and rice. These are simple things but they reduce the high fever and clear the infection from the brain. Modern medicine and TCM used together is the most effective treatment.

Menopause

Although this is a natural change, it does not always go smoothly. Women can suffer from hot flushes, depression, migraine, headaches, or loss of calcium, leading to osteoporosis. The diagnosis in TCM is likely to be an imbalance between liver and kidneys, with weakness in the kidneys and blood deficiency.

Acupuncture can often help, but in the more serious cases herbal medicine is usually more effective in restoring the body's internal balance and the balance of the hormones. Chinese angelica root, raw and cooked rehmannia, peony root and thorowax root are commonly used. These work well and do not produce the side-effects sometimes involved in hormonal treatment.

Menstrual problems

In general, these are diagnosed as an imbalance of liver, spleen and kidney. Excessive blood loss is ascribed to heat in the blood. Late, scanty and painful periods are due to cold in the blood. Acupuncture and moxibustion are often very effective in coping with these common problems. Diet is also important, and heavy periods, diagnosed as a disease pattern involving heat, would include advice to avoid 'hot' food. Menstrual irregularities caused by cold conditions would involve avoiding 'cold' food (see Chapter 8).

Migraine

A variety of symptoms are associated with this distressing condition. The headaches may be preceded by flashing lights, blurred vision and other visual disturbances such as an 'aura' caused by temporary narrowing of the blood vessels to the brain. Immediately afterwards the arteries open up, allowing a gush of blood to the brain and causing a severe throbbing pain on one side of the head.

Not all migraines follow the same pattern. Some sufferers experience numbness and tingling in the arms, or feelings of exhaustion, and extreme sensitivity to light. In TCM migraine is caused by excessive stagnation of energy in the liver and gallbladder which invades the stomach. The pain above the eyes, or flashing lights with pain in the forehead or sides of the head, indicate involvement of the channels from the liver. The nausea is caused by liver invasion of the stomach.

Treatment concentrates on strengthening and tonifying the stomach, reducing the tension in the liver, and moving the qi from the liver and gallbladder. Ginseng, poria, ginger, and Chinese date would be used for the stomach; skullcap, thorowax root and strong purging herbs such as Chinese gentian for the liver; with acupuncture for the headaches. This treatment has an encouraging success rate. Acupuncture is often very effective; acupressure can achieve the same effect for people who are squeamish about needles, but herbal medicines can also be prescribed. A combination of these methods can often be highly successful. Chinese meditation techniques can also help.

Morning sickness

In China a pregnant woman suffering from mild morning sickness would be advised to eat warm foods such as fresh ginger, and to avoid cold foods. Serious sickness would be considered a weakness of the stomach and an overstrained liver, with too much heat in the body. Acupuncture can help, but it must be stressed that this should only be carried out by a fully qualified and highly experienced practitioner. The needles must be used with great care, and only on the arms and legs. In the wrong hands, acupuncture could possibly trigger miscarriage.

Ginger tea is an effective remedy, easily made at home. It has been used for centuries in China and is now being hailed in the West as an effective home-made remedy for sickness. Slice 25–50 g/1–2 oz fresh ginger into 575 ml/1 pint water, bring to the boil and simmer for 10 minutes. Sweeten if desired.

Mosquito bites

Although painful and sore, causing swellings and intense irritation, these are usually more of a nuisance than a danger. If you have been travelling in the tropics, however, a mosquito bite could have more serious implications. A female mosquito can spread malaria (see page 166) if it has previously bitten someone whose blood is infected by the parasite which causes the disease. Every year, around 1,500 people in Britain develop malaria, after returning from a trip abroad, and a few cases are fatal. Because of climatic changes some cases of malaria have been recorded in people who were bitten here although fortunately these are very rare. Anyone who develops a feverish headache accompanied by sweating after a mosquito bite should seek medical advice. The disease can have an incubation period of up to ten months. Serious bites are treated with herbs to detoxify the blood. Palm oil, easily bought at an oriental supermarket, is good to use on mild bites.

Mouth ulcers

These small round or oval ulcers with a yellowish edge can appear for no apparent reason, and recur regularly. They are very painful and can take about a week to clear. They may indicate that the sufferer is run down, or they may be stress-related.

A TCM doctor sees them as caused by either heat in the heart, heat in the stomach or weakness of the kidneys. If they occur on the tongue, the cause is heat in the heart, or sometimes the spleen. Ulcers around the gums are caused by heat in the stomach. If they are all over the mouth, and constantly recur, this is caused by the kidneys. People who suffer from mouth ulcers should avoid spicy foods, deep-fried foods or acidic fruit like citrus fruit. Plenty of greens should be included in the diet, the bowels should be kept open, and plenty of sleep is also recommended.

If you have a bad problem, consult a TCM doctor and he will prescribe according to the symptoms. Rhubarb, rehmannia root, lily root, or the Chinese remedy Six Rehmannia Pills are also used. Herbs made into powder can be applied direct to the ulcers to make them heal more quickly.

Moxibustion

Although Chinese in origin and regularly used by TCM doctors, this technique of burning the artemisia herb (the common mugwort) on the end of an acupuncture needle to apply heat into the channels to tone and regulate the flow of qi, is even more popular in Japan, and it is from the Japanese word for the process that moxibustion gets its name.

The moxa 'wool' is actually the dried or shredded leaves of the plant, and it can either be twisted on to the acupuncture needle after it is inserted or used in a paper tube and held above the appropriate acupoint by the practitioner. A pleasant, warm sensation is produced as the needle heats or the heat from the moxa tube penetrates the skin. It is a very effective way of both warming the body and drawing out infections.

Multiple sclerosis

MS, as it is usually called, results from damage to the myelin sheaths surrounding the nerve fibres of the central nervous system. The cause of this is not known, it may be a genetic disorder, or caused by a virus. About one person in every 2,000 is affected, with a higher proportion of women. It may begin as tingling, numbness or weakness affecting an arm or leg or one side of the body. Sometimes symptoms include double vision, or blurring of the sight. The attack may happen only once and never recur, but in most cases it runs a course of relapses and remissions over many years. Weakness, difficulty in walking, slurred speech and loss of bladder control are some of the attendant problems.

The TCM diagnosis is a general weakness of the whole body, especially the kidneys, which causes the central nervous system to malfunction and results in wastage of the muscles. Acupuncture can be used to improve the circulation, stimulate the nervous system and help the muscles. Herbs will deal with kidney and stomach weakness, revitalizing them to stop deterioration. When the kidneys are weak, they cannot process the nutrients in the body, and the central nervous system is starved. Medicine will tonify the kidneys and spleen.

MS is a serious problem. Treatment should begin as soon as it is diagnosed. The earlier it is caught, the better the prognosis. The problems associated with the complaint

– kidney and bladder infections and blurred vision, etc. – respond well to TCM treatment, and the progress of the MS itself can be controlled. Therapy is long-term, but it is one of the conditions where TCM has had much more success than modern medicine (see case histories, page 65).

Mumps

One of the most common ailments of childhood, mumps is caused by a viral infection in the saliva glands. It may only affect one side of the face, but often spreads to the opposite gland a day or two later. Along with swollen glands there may be earache, particularly when eating. Although adult men who catch mumps may suffer swelling and inflammation of the testicles, this rarely leads to sterility, contrary to common belief. In women, inflammation of the ovaries can cause abdominal pain, but again, is unlikely to result in permanent damage.

Mumps is infectious and often occurs in epidemics, particularly in spring and summer. TCM regards it as an invasion of wind damp heat which has become lodged in the facial area and therefore causes the painful swelling of the glands. Herbs like honeysuckle flowers, isatis root, dandelion, skullcap root or rhubarb can all be used in the treatment.

Muscular dystrophy

This is a genetic disorder, leading to progressive wasting of the muscles. The Duchenne type begins in childhood, affecting boys between four and ten years old. It starts with a weakness in the legs, the child may walk on tiptoe all the time, or start to waddle, and be unable to climb stairs. It is progressively debilitating, causing curvature of the spine, and there is no cure although physiotherapy and other forms of assistance can be given. TCM works on the kidneys, spleen and stomach to help digestion so that the body can absorb nutrients to help muscles. The Six Gentlemen and acupuncture will be given to stimulate the muscles and help the circulation to the tissues (see case history, page 67).

Myocarditis

Another condition where TCM and Western medicine can usefully combine to increase the patient's recovery markedly. Chinese medicine will treat the kidneys as well as the heart itself, because the theory is that the heart is the organ of fire, and the kidneys – the water organ – must balance the fire. Therefore, tonifying the kidneys to prevent any further weakness can balance the heat in the heart. Herbs such as lily root, ginseng and rehmannia root are commonly used in such cases.

Nausea and vomiting

Feeling sick and vomiting are symptoms, not diseases. They may result from overeating or car sickness, a simple upset tummy or many different causes. If the condition persists, and there is no apparent reason for it, seek medical advice.

TCM treatment usually involves making the stomach qi descend. Acupuncture is also effective. A successful acupoint for stopping nausea and vomiting is located, with the palm upwards, along the arm from the wrist fold, and between the two tendons.

Nephritis

Inflammation of the kidneys, often following a streptococcal infection of the throat, flu or tonsillitis. It usually affects children. The kidneys cease to function, leading to raised blood pressure, vomiting or sometimes fits. The urine is scanty, and has a smoky or a bloody tinge. Fluid retention causes tissue swelling around the eyes, and repeated attacks can lead to chronic kidney failure.

Modern medicine treats with antibiotics and diuretic drugs. In TCM, the illness is connected with the lungs, spleen and kidneys, and all three will be treated. There is a blockage of the lungs, causing oedema. Acute nephritis often follows, and Chinese doctors regard it as the heat from those conditions invading the lungs. Oedema can also be connected with a weakness of the spleen, tiredness and swollen limbs, but some kinds also involve kidney deficiency, so the overall treatment has to be carefully chosen. Bamboo leaves, thistle or water plantain and rhubarb are effective. If it becomes chronic, tonic herbs will include Six Rehmannia Pills and Return Spleen Pills.

Any possibility of a kidney infection must be checked immediately with a GP.

Nettle rash

The medical name for this unpleasant condition is urticaria. It is also sometimes called hives. Raised red patches or weals appear on the skin, causing swelling and intense itching. It may be due to a food allergy, and can sometimes be caused by a reaction to aspirin. Stress is also a contributory factor in some cases, and often makes the condition worse. In bad cases, the eyes, lips and throat can swell dramatically. If this happens, seek medical help immediately. When the condition is red and hot it is attributed to heat and wind; in cases where there is a cold white rash, it is due to cold and wind. The lung channels must be opened to expel the wind and calm the body. Schizonepeta or ledebouriella root might be used.

Neuralgia

Acute nerve pains in the head or face are diagnosed in TCM as wind, fire and heat in the channels connected with the liver and gallbladder. Acupuncture will open the channels and herbs prescribed to clear wind and heat internally.

Nose and throat ailments

The nose is directly dominated by the lungs. Treatment will be through the lung channel or the lungs themselves. Sneezing or a runny nose is a weakness caused by wind and cold in the lung. Throat problems can also be due to a blockage in the lung. Mulberry leaf, plantain seed, peppermint, honeysuckle flowers or skullcap will be used.

Nose-bleeds are the result of heat in the blood. In the case of women who have nose-bleeds during menstrual periods, the problem is considered to be blood rising instead of descending. Fresh herbs are the most effective cure for this condition, rehmannia, peony root and thistle being the ones most commonly used.

Obesity

A person is considered obese when they weigh 20 per cent or more above the average for their height and build. Causes can be very complicated. The most common may be overeating and inactivity, but many obese people have a metabolism problem or a hormone imbalance. TCM considers obesity is due to the spleen and kidneys. Sufferers have too much phlegm or dampness in the body. Trying to lose weight through diet will have short-term results. A 'cold' food diet will further weaken the spleen. Sufferers should eat healthy food in moderation (see Chapter 8).

A TCM doctor will aim to strengthen the deficient organs. Acupuncture can help. Herbal medicine treatment is complicated in these cases, and very individual, but it can certainly be an aid. Once the harmony of the body is restored to balance, the metabolism will process food properly, and excess weight should no longer be a problem, provided the correct foods are taken in moderate quantities.

Oedema

In Western medicine this is a heart, liver or kidney problem, but in TCM it is also related to the spleen and lung. It is caused because the body cannot get rid of excess water. The spleen is important because, in TCM, it processes the food and the blood and transforms the dampness. The lung can also be responsible if there is a blockage.

If a kidney deficiency is diagnosed it will be treated by warming and tonifying to restore the balance. Herbs used include aconite, dried ginger and water plantain to prevent production of further dampness. For the spleen, ginseng, codonopsis root, poria and white atractylodes tuber would be prescribed. The lung herbs are intended to send the lung energy downwards, and the herbs used here would be cinnamon twigs and ephedra.

In TCM curing oedema is not simply a case of taking diuretic drugs. They are not the answer as the system becomes dependent upon them, and once you stop taking them the body fills up with water again. If they are taken long-term they can cause other damage. TCM treats the cause, not the symptoms.

Osteoarthritis

The result of wear and tear on the joints, damaging the cartilage between the bones. The joints may become swollen and deformed, mainly at the hips, knees, knuckles and spine. This condition can be successfully treated by TCM if it is caught in the early stages. It is seen as mainly due to weakness in the kidney and the liver, plus a lack of energy causing stagnation in the blood. It is important to keep warm. Pubescent angelica root, ledebouriella root, or timos-pora stem, cinnamon twigs and mulberry twigs will warm the channels of the body and the blood, improving circulation and nourishing the joints. This helps to stop further deterioration in advanced cases, and can sometimes bring about a cure if treatment begins at the very first signs of the disease. When the joints are badly damaged, they cannot be restored.

Osteoporosis

One of the hazards for post-menopausal women, this is caused by loss of calcium in the bones, which become progressively weaker, thinner and more brittle, and can break very easily, particularly at the pelvis or the wrist. The condition can sometimes begin to affect people as early as in their twenties.

Loss of bone mass leads to the spine gradually becoming shorter and more curved, causing loss of height and hunched shoulders, 'dowager's hump'. Exercise is very important, even a leisurely daily walk is therapeutic, and the gentle Chinese exercise system of tai qi can be extremely effective. It will boost the emotional and mental energies as well as helping the patient to function normally.

In TCM, as the kidneys dominate the bones, so osteoporosis is the result of a kidney deficiency. If bones become decalcified, it is through lack of nourishment to the kidneys. The treatment is concentrated on tonifying herbs. Drynaria tuber, cibot rhizome and eucommia bark might be prescribed, depending on the severity of the problem. It must be caught in the early stages, to prevent further damage or slow down deterioration. As the kidneys lie deep in the body, they are not easy to tonify quickly, so treatment must be long-term.

Ovulation problems

Abdominal pain during the menstrual cycle can be treated by balancing the liver and blood. Problems like infertility caused through irregular ovulation are treated through the kidneys, balancing the blood and qi and nourishing the blood. This can increase fertility. TCM is particularly successful in treating 'women's problems'. Moxibustion is often extremely effective and several patent medicines which can be bought over the counter from a TCM pharmacy have been in use for generations. These can be obtained from Chinese herbal shops, and the herbalist will advise on the best one for each particular client. Angelica Pills or Women's Precious Pills can be useful.

Palpitations

May be caused by nervous tension or even drinking too much coffee, but can result from heart problems. If palpitations recur frequently, your GP will arrange for hospital tests. A rapid heartbeat, called tachycardia, can be caused by an overactive thyroid. It particularly affects anxious people. Elderly people or alcoholics often have an irregular heartbeat, which may be due to disease of the heart valves.

Everyone experiences an extra heartbeat at times, or the sensation that the heart 'missed a beat'. This is often due to anxiety, but if it happens regularly it may be a symptom of a heart disorder. When a serious heart condition is suspected, orthodox treatment at a Western hospital, with ECG tests, is vital. These would automatically be carried out in a TCM hospital in China, where all the modern diagnostic equipment is used.

Chinese doctors regard palpitations as evidence of a deficiency of the heart and the heart blood: medicine would include lilyturf root, asparagus root, wild jujube seeds, dogwood fruit or fleece-flower stem, which nourish the heart and calm palpitations. Acupuncture is good for palpitations which are not due to physical reasons.

Parkinson's disease

Slowness in moving and muscular stiffness are among the first symptoms of this illness, which rarely affects those under the age of fifty. It is relatively common in older people, affecting one in every 1,000, and men slightly more than women. As it progresses, the muscles of the face stiffen, walking becomes increasingly difficult, and speech may be affected. In most cases, a tremor in the limbs is present. The disease is caused by degeneration of nerve cells in the brain responsible for controlling movement, and a shortage of dopamine, a substance which is thought to be a neurotransmitter.

Patients consulting a TCM doctor will be treated for a liver and kidney problem, with deficiency of blood and kidney yin. This leads to lack of nourishment to the brain through internal 'wind', making the body shake like a tree in a gale. The liver and kidney must be nourished to increase the body fluids. Some milder cases can be helped, but there is a better outcome with younger people who are new sufferers than in long-term cases with older patients. Acupuncture will help and will be given in tandem with herbal medicine. There will not be a complete cure. Fleece-flower root, mulberry root and uncaria stem are good to extinguish the wind, and herbs to move the blood and nourish the liver are peony buds and white peony root. One herb that is commonly used is gastrodia tuber, which nourishes the brain, blood and kidneys and stops the shaking.

Peptic ulcer

A problem seen in TCM as often involving weakness of the spleen, stagnation of stomach qi and stagnation of the liver which overstrains the stomach. Liver stagnation also causes depression and anxiety, so there can be an emotional aspect. Treatment depends on the severity of the condition. If it is mild and in the early stages, the medicine used would be intended to clear the heat, move the stagnation and help the digestion. When the case is long-term, a spleen weakness is also involved. In advanced stages, there can be internal bleeding which must also be stopped.

Sufferers need to be taught to relax and watch their diet. Tea, coffee and alcohol should be avoided, particularly when the stomach is empty. Foods which the Chinese classify as 'cold' (such as salads), are not good for people with ulcers. The burning pain can be helped by dandelion or dandelion juice, but in a very painful case, corydalis tuber would be used. For too much acid, squid bone is effective. Notoginseng can aid the healing of the ulcer, because it can help the growth of tissue.

Phlebitis

TCM doctors say that heat and poison in the blood vessels are causing a blockage. The heat must first be cleared, the blood cooled and the poisons flushed out with peony bark, saffron, lovage tuber, Chinese golden thread or rhubarb root. This condition is slow to respond to herbal medicine but the condition can be alleviated in many cases, and sometimes cured.

Pimples and spots

These are quite normal at puberty when the metabolism is altering, and poisons come out in the skin. When spots come out excessively, the heat in the blood and stomach must be cooled. Herbal tea made of honeysuckle, chrysanthemum or dandelion will clear the heat in simple cases. Severe cases involve medicine made from skullcap, rhubarb, even gypsum. Fresh rehmannia is also effective.

In China, patent herbal creams can be bought over the counter but they are not available in Britain. A reasonable substitute is to cleanse the skin with fresh watermelon, which is very cooling. Either watermelon or cucumber is good for the skin and makes a simple, inexpensive but beneficial beauty treatment.

Pink eye

Another name for conjunctivitis. Caused by wind-heat in the liver channels, allowing a build-up of poisons in the body. A herbal decoction will help, or, in bad cases, the herb will be steamed. Cultivated or wild chrysanthemum flowers, bamboo leaves or violet would be used. They are cooked and the cooled water can be used to bathe the eyes.

Pneumonia

A viral or bacterial infection usually causes pneumonia, and although the viral form can be dangerous, especially in vulnerable elderly people or the young, bacterial pneumonia is the more serious health hazard. It may be the final cause of death in cancer victims or the very old.

If only one lobe of lung is affected, it is known as acute lobar pneumonia. It develops rapidly, causing fever, rapid breathing and a dry, persistent cough. Bronchopneumonia involves patchy inflammation which can be on one or both lungs, and double pneumonia simply means that both lungs are affected. In TCM the diagnosis will be heat and phlegm in the lung, mainly due to a wind heat or wind cold invasion.

Treatment varies according to the stage. In the early days, when there is coughing, fever and chest pain, it is treated in a similar way to bronchitis or flu. When there is blood in the phlegm, the heat must be cleared. Skullcap, fritillary bulb, houttuynia, lepidium seed or peach kernel may be used. A GP must be consulted quickly.

Poliomyelitis

Familiar thirty years ago in Britain, fortunately uncommon now, this is an acute viral infection causing degeneration of the spinal cord and consequent paralysis. Acupuncture can sometimes revitalize the nerve cells which have suffered damage. Herbs are used to nourish nerves, blood and qi.

Pregnancy

TCM doctors advise pregnant women to relax and follow tranquil pursuits, to eat foods rich in calcium and fibre and to avoid constipation. It is very important to move around, to prevent qi and blood stagnation which can lead to oedema or high blood pressure. An active pregnancy also makes labour easier. Pregnant Chinese women with high blood pressure can be given herbal medicine. *Always consult a GP before taking any medicines in pregnancy.*

Premenstrual syndrome

The feelings of depression, aggression, bloatedness, headaches, pain and water retention experienced by victims of PMS are usually caused by an imbalance of the liver, kidneys and spleen. TCM considers menstruation to be the monthly release of an overflowing blood reservoir, and stagnation which interferes with this process causes problems like PMS. Acupuncture and herbal medicine can stimulate the liver, and diet therapy is often useful. Chinese angelica, white peony, skullcap, and poria or sometimes green mandarin orange peel can be very effective.

Prolapse

According to TCM theory, the prolapse of organs is caused by a deficiency of the qi in the middle of the body. This is a weakness often experienced by older people, and a well-known medicine to tonify the spleen, called Central Qi Pills, will be prescribed. Astragalus, thorowax root and cimicifuga tuber make up this prescription. The individual treatment will depend upon the actual organ involved.

Prostate problems

Enlargement of the prostate gland is a common problem in older men and can easily be corrected by surgery. For those who would prefer to avoid an operation, TCM treatment may be able to provide the answer. The dampness in the body has to be eradicated and the qi moved. This is a complicated treatment, but plantain seed, water plantain, cinnamon bark and corktree bark will be used (see case history, page 68).

Psoriasis

Chinese herbal treatments for this distressing skin condition are undergoing clinical trials at several hospitals and the outlook is extremely encouraging. The raised, red scaly patches can appear anywhere on the body, but most often affect the knees or elbows. The cause is unknown and it is uncommon before the age of ten. It usually affects both sides of the body and often makes the nails on fingers and toes become thickened and pitted. Psoriasis responds well to treatment by individual TCM doctors, although they emphasize that some cases are very stubborn. Relatively mild cases can respond in two or three months. Serious cases take much longer, and a cure cannot be guaranteed. The condition is often due to a blood heat syndrome.

Quinsy

Caused by an abscess forming behind one of the tonsils during an attack of tonsillitis. It may cause difficulty in swallowing and speaking and the pain is likely to be worse on the affected side of the throat.

A TCM doctor will treat quinsy as heat and fire poison in the blood. Strong herbs are used to treat the inflammation of the tonsils and surrounding tissues, including Chinese golden thread, skullcap, pigeon peas, dandelion and forsythia fruit.

Raynaud's disease

This extremely painful and serious complaint takes its name from the French physician who identified and researched the condition. It affects people who are hypersensitive to cold. The hands and feet suddenly turn pale and numb. In severe cases, they take on a bluish tinge and there is a burning pain. About 5 per cent of people in Britain suffer from this disorder at some stage in their lives. It usually affects women more than men. In China it is equally familiar, and is regularly treated in TCM hospitals. If caught in the early stages, there is a good prognosis, but in advanced stages (fortunately rare) gangrene may develop and amputation may be necessary. Cinnamon twigs and Chinese angelica are effective in this treatment (see case history, page 69).

Restlessness

The kind experienced during the menopause, or through PMT or anxiety following an illness is considered in TCM to be due to heat in the heart caused by blood or yin deficiency. Some cases are due to internal heat. If the problem is serious, medicine to calm the heart will be given. This is a symptom, not a disease, and the doctor will try to discover what is causing the problem and treat accordingly. Lilyturf root and lotus seed sprouts made into tea will nourish the yin and the blood.

Rheumatism

Mainly wind heat and damp in the body. Corktree bark, achyran-thus root and coix lachryma joba are good for acute rheumatism. Chronic rheumatism is chronic qi stagnation and herbs will be prescribed which move the blood and the qi. There is a good prognosis for cases that are seen early. In later stages, medicine can help to reduce the swelling.

Rheumatoid arthritis

Many patients of TCM doctors in Britain report pain relief and all-round improvement after a course of treatment. Treatment is similar to rheumatism, but there is sometimes a lot of coldness in the body too. Herbs vary considerably in individual cases, but one effective herb is *Tripterytium wilfordii*. Acupuncture is effective for stopping pain in joints and helping movement. There is also a medicine which can be applied externally. As a home remedy, to ease discomfort, powdered rhubarb mixed with sesame oil helps the swelling for both forms of arthritis. Chronic arthritis can be helped by herbal plasters, which are generally available from doctors, (see case history, page 70).

Rubella (German measles)

Seldom serious, except if caught by an expectant mother in the early months of pregnancy, rubella is highly infectious, but once it is over, the patient usually has immunity for life. It starts as a mild fever, then the glands become swollen behind the ears and an orangy-pink rash appears on the face and spreads to the rest of the body.

It is possible for girls to have an injection against rubella at thirteen years of age. Any woman who contracts the disease during the first three months of pregnancy should discuss the matter with the ante-natal doctor. A termination may be advised.

Chinese traditional theory sees it as an external wind-heat invasion or wind cold. The treatment to clear the wind and heat includes ledebouriella root and schizonepeta. Mulberry leaves, or honeysuckle or chrysanthemum flowers will be used where the problem is diagnosed as heat. When wind cold is diagnosed, cinnamon twigs will be added.

Schizophrenia

This is a serious mental disorder which usually strikes between the teens and twenties, often affecting very bright and promising young people. They may suffer delusions of persecution, for example that messages are coming through the television, or that their minds are being controlled by some hidden force. They may hear voices instructing them to violent or bizarre acts, and suffer from irrational fears. TCM considers this a problem of imbalance between heart, kidneys and liver. The spirit, the shen which normally resides in the heart, is floating and not controlled. To calm the shen, the heart and kidneys will be nourished and the liver soothed. In order to maintain physical and mental balance, the vulnerable spirit must be housed safely, and if this is not the case, then the heart must be too weak to do its job properly.

One well-known remedy is Emperor Tea Pills which work in unison with the Free and Easy Wanderer. In China, treatment includes acupuncture and several metals: cinnabar and even gold are used regularly and are both very effective. A common technique in TCM hospitals is to make a small incision in the skin of the arm and insert a tiny piece of gold, in rather the same way that hormone implants are carried out in this country. The process cannot be done by TCM doctors practising in Britain, as they are not allowed to carry out even small surgical operations. There is an old, and still widely held belief in China that pure gold will calm the spirit and calm the evil in the body. Gold is greatly prized for its therapeutic properties. Babies often wear either gold or silver bracelets, anklets or chains, not just because the metals protect the shen, but because they are considered to be a good monitor of general health. A silver bracelet will change colour according to the chemicals excreted by the pores, and acts as a barometer to the child's condition. In China, convulsions can be treated by boiling a piece of pure gold, a ring or a similar piece of jewellery, and giving the child the warm water to drink. It may be that some extract from the gold seeps into the water.

Sciatica

Begins when the sciatic nerve is irritated or compressed at its root at the base of the spine, causing severe shooting pains which will run down the back and outside the leg from the thigh to the foot. It can be caused by a slipped disc, ankylosing spondylitis or osteoarthritis. It can come on suddenly, after something as simple as a twisting movement of the body, and it is worse on bending, sneezing or coughing.

TCM sees this as damp heat stagnation in the gallbladder meridian or in the urinary bladder meridian. If the condition is chronic, cold and blood stagnation are the cause. Acupuncture can be very successful.

Seasickness

Peppermint oil on the temples and the roof of the mouth below the nasal passages will help, as will chewing a piece of fresh ginger. The wrist-bands which can be bought at any chemist's can be very useful in making boat journeys a pleasant experience for bad sailors. They exert gentle, constant pressure on the acupoint, another small advance for which the West can thank traditional Chinese medicine. Pressure on the acupoint 5 cm/2 inches down from the wrist (palm upward) may come in useful as a do-it-yourself treatment if seasickness comes on unexpectedly.

Shingles

The cause of shingles is the chickenpox virus which can lie dormant at the root of a nerve for many years, long after the patient has forgotten even having the disease. It can be reactivated by stress, or sometimes by contact with a child who has chickenpox. A red, blistered skin rash preceded by intense, searing pain can affect any part of the body, including the eyes. The rash sometimes forms a semicircle around the waist, giving rise to the old belief that if the spots meet in the middle, the victim is doomed. Painful and unpleasant though shingles can be, it is not fatal. The medical name, *Herpes Zoster*, comes from the Greek words *herpes* (to creep), and *zoster* (girdle).

The blisters usually heal quite quickly, but the nerve pain can go on for months. If the facial nerve is affected, the face may be temporarily paralysed, and if the optic nerve is affected, the cornea can be seriously damaged, endangering the sight. See a doctor as soon as possible if shingles affect the area near the eyes. In TCM, it will probably be diagnosed as heat and damp in the gallbladder and the liver channels. Herbal medicine, including oriental wormwood and Chinese gentian, is usually effective.

Shoulder stiffness
See Frozen shoulder.

Sinus problems
Sinusitis is caused by inflammation of the mucous membranes in the sinuses, the air-filled spaces in the bones of the face. Symptoms are a blocked-up nose, a nasal tone in the speech, and sometimes a headache over one or both eyes, usually worse in the mornings, when lying down or bending forwards. Normally mucus is channelled through the tiny air ducts to the nose, but during colds the ducts can become congested and when the mucus builds up, the sinuses become inflamed. Hay fever can also cause sinusitis, and allergy to dust or tobacco smoke can result in chronic cases. There can also be a greenish-yellow or bloody discharge from the nose.

A TCM physician will see the condition as mainly connected with a lung qi deficiency and with damp heat. Peppermint, honeysuckle, fritillary bulb, tangerine peel and xanthium fruit are all helpful.

Slipped disc
The vertebrae at the top of the spine are separated from each other by discs of cartilage which cushion them from impact. The discs have a fibrous outer casing surrounding a soft, pulpy centre, and when the casing is damaged, the pulpy centre will either bulge out or burst, causing a slipped, or prolapsed, disc.

This can irritate other ligaments of the outer membrane of the spinal cord, or may constrict a spinal nerve. The pain may be severe, dull or aching, either at the site of the problem or elsewhere along the area served by the affected nerve. There may also be muscle spasm, nerve irritation or numbness in the leg or foot. If the problem recurs, the weak ligaments can be helped by tonifying the kidneys and strengthening the muscles. Herbs include cinnamon bark, wolfberry and eucommia bark (see case history, page 72).

Spastic colon

See also Irritable Bowel Syndrome. This condition often responds positively to TCM treatment. The spleen and liver must be balanced, the qi moved, cold cleared and the blood nourished. Cinnamon twigs with white peony root, astragalus, fresh ginger and Chinese black bait can be used.

Sperm disorders

A TCM doctor will first check to see if an infection or tumour is involved, or if the testicles are undescended. These conditions must be treated first. When a low sperm count is the problem, herbs to strengthen and tonify the kidneys will improve this condition. A wide variety of herbs can be used to help, but the cause may vary from kidney essence deficiency to a deficiency of kidney yang or kidney yin, with a different form of treatment in each case (see case history; page 60).

Spots

Caused by heat in the stomach. Sufferers should avoid 'hot' foods. Chinese golden thread, skullcap or rhubarb can help. Dandelion or liquorice will cool the heat.

Stress

It is important to identify the source of the stress and try to tackle it, to eat a good diet and to get plenty of sleep, and always find time to relax. Meditation will help (see Chapter 9), and so can acupuncture. Herbal medicines will induce calm. Thorowax root, peony root and schizandra fruit may be prescribed.

Stroke

TCM defines two kinds of stroke, of the head and of the heart. A head stroke is called a wind stroke and can occasionally be fatal or leave victims partly paralysed. It happens when the blood supply to the brain is disturbed or insufficient and can vary in severity and symptoms. There may be sudden loss of movement or speech, dizziness, blurred vision, sudden heaviness in the limbs or feelings of numbness, and a loss of consciousness. If symptoms last for more than twenty-four hours, a full stroke has occurred. Sometimes they wear off after a few hours, in which case the condition is called a transient ischaemic attack. One in three strokes is fatal, and, depending on the extent of damage, survivors may be left with impairment of speech, movement or ability to read.

The TCM treatment involves nourishing the liver and the kidneys, to move the blood and open the channel to clear the wind. Herbal prescriptions are complicated and depend on the severity of the stroke, but a very effective medicine involves lovage tuber which is said to dissolve or prevent blood clots in the brain. It can be made into an injection and given intravenously.

After a stroke, acupuncture can often be extremely helpful in treating paralysis and aiding the recovery of those with speech difficulties. The earlier it is started, the more effective and the speedier the response will be. Where the damage is of very long standing, recovery is likely to be slow, and may not be effective.

Sweating

Excessive sweating is often embarrassing, but usually harmless. It often begins with the hormonal changes at puberty, and becomes less of a problem as the sufferer grows up, but occasionally it can last a lifetime. Good hygiene is important, but if the problem is really serious, an operation can be carried out to reduce the number of sweat glands in the armpit by removing some of the skin.

Abnormally profuse sweating, called spontaneous sweating, is regarded in TCM as a deficiency of the qi, and in particular the 'defensive' qi. It may occur in old people, or in a patient who is recovering from illness and is still very weak. Night sweats are due to yin deficiency.

The treatment in the first type will be to tonify the qi, in the second type the yin must be nourished. For yin deficiency, peony, corktree bark and lilyturf root are used. For qi deficiency, astragalus and ledebouriella are used.

Tapeworms

Tapeworms can be transmitted in infected meat or fish which has not been properly cooked. The embryonic parasite develops a head which fastens itself into the wall of the small intestine, and then grows into a long, segmented worm which feeds on the predigested contents. Segments which contain thousands of embryos occasionally break off and appear in faeces. The symptoms are itching around the anus and occasional abdominal pain. There is also likely to be some weight loss, but not undue hunger, unless the person is already suffering from malnutrition.

Sometimes these can cause a complete blockage of the intestine, in which case herbal medicine would be used to calm the tapeworms before killing and expelling them. Afterwards – or sometimes even before – the TCM doctor will attempt to tonify the energy of the spleen, to strengthen the body, repair the damage and prevent reinfection.

There are many medicines which can be used. Among the most common are pumpkin seeds, followed by betel nut, followed by a purgative medicine such as rhubarb.

TATT (Tired All The Time syndrome)

Everyone goes through periods of feeling worn out, lacking in energy and generally run down at some point in life. The feeling may be caused by overwork or general stress, in which case it usually wears off when the contributory cause is tackled. If it becomes a chronic condition, and the victim wakes every morning feeling drained and tired, unable to concentrate or to take an interest in events, it is sometimes diagnosed as TATT. More patients consult a doctor complaining of these symptoms than for anything else, and the contributory factors can be varied, from an underlying physical illness to depression.

Reading the pulse and examining the tongue will help the TCM doctor to decide whether the condition is emotional or physical, and he will take a full case history to see whether there are psychological or environmental factors which need to be looked at. Chronic tiredness can be a symptom of premenstrual tension or the menopause, or it may involve some other hormonal imbalance, perhaps an underactive thyroid, or Addison's Disease, in which the body has too little adrenalin.

If the patient is just tired, TCM diagnoses a qi deficiency; if tired and feeling cold, yang deficiency; if tired and hot, a yin deficiency. It is vital to make the right diagnosis, as treatment varies accordingly. Ginseng can be effective for some types of tiredness, but it must be administered carefully. Other herbs are usually needed as well.

Teeth grinding

Many people grind their teeth in their sleep, possibly because of anxiety, but sometimes also as the result of something as simple as misaligned or missing teeth, or an uneven bite. If teeth grinding persists, it can eventually lead to disorders of the joint of the jaw, and arthritis can develop. TCM believes that teeth grinding is sometimes caused by heat in the spleen and the stomach, which comes out in the evenings.

In the case of a child it may indicate the presence of some kind of parasite in the intestines. If tests show that it is not the cause, the child will be given treatment designed to cool the heat in the spleen. Medicines might include Chinese yam, skullcap, or even a little Chinese golden thread or lotus seeds.

Tendon disorders

The tendons are controlled by the liver, according to TCM theory. Therefore, if the liver is nourished, weak or damaged, the tendons will get stronger. But even someone with a very strong liver can sustain a tendon injury through a sporting mishap, in which case the doctor will attempt to improve the circulation of the blood and the qi to stop the internal bleeding and clear the bruise inside. Herbs can also be used to clear the cold and damp which cause swollen tendons in people with chronic arthritis.

Tennis elbow

Inflammation of the tendon which joins the muscles of the forearm to the lower end of the upper arm bone (the humerus). The muscles at the back of the forearm flex the fingers and wrists, and they are all connected to the same point on the outer side of the humerus. Not surprisingly, in view of the muscles' constant use, inflammation can sometimes result, causing extreme tenderness and pain down the forearm and up to the shoulder.

Any repetitive action – typing, working at a supermarket checkout, or repeated lifting – can cause this condition, as well as playing tennis frequently. If it persists, and is caused by an aspect of the victim's work which they are unable to avoid, a GP may prescribe anti-inflammatory drugs or cortisone injections.

A TCM physician will say it is caused by cold and damp in the elbow region. Treatment with herbal medicines including cinnamon twigs, mulberry twigs, angelica root and white ginger can be very effective, as can acupuncture combined with moxibustion.

Threadworms

Threadworms are a common problem in China. The treatment given in TCM is similar to that for tapeworms. These tiny white worms, sometimes called pinworms, which look just like small piece of thread, can cause intense itching in and around the anus. They infect the large intestine and are expelled in the faeces. At night, the female threadworms emerge to lay up to 10,000 eggs in the surrounding area of the anus. The eggs live for up to three weeks and are highly infectious.

In children, the itching causes the child to scratch, transferring the worms to his hands and under his fingernails. Later, if he puts his fingers in his mouth or touches food, they can be swallowed and reach the intestine where the whole cycle begins again. Hygiene is very important. Hands should be washed and the nails thoroughly scrubbed before each meal, and each time the child uses the lavatory, and the seams of underclothing should be carefully ironed because worms can also lie concealed in the folds of material.

Several herbs are effective, particularly quisqualis, whose seed should be fried or toasted and then chewed. (This remedy is toxic unless taken in small quantities and the dose must be precisely calculated. A TCM doctor will prescribe the right amount.)

Thrush

This is caused by a yeastlike fungus called Candida albicans or Monilia, which thrives in warm, moist areas of the body. The problem is also known as Candida. It can be present for a long time before it is detected, as it does not cause symptoms in the early stages. Recurrent attacks are common.

The thrush organism lives on the skin, and attacks can flare up easily, particularly in the warm, moist skin folds. It is worse in people who are overweight, and can affect the groin, armpits and the skin under the breasts, making the affected areas red, itchy and sore.

Thrush in the vulva and vagina is very common and can be extremely difficult to cure completely. It causes itching and soreness with a white, curdy discharge. It is not necessarily sexually transmitted, but a partner may develop the infection with redness and soreness on the end of the penis and under the foreskin, and reinfection can be passed back and forward between one partner and the other. It is advisable not to wear tights or clinging jeans if you are prone to thrush. It is best to wear undergarments made of natural fibres which allow the skin to breathe.

A TCM doctor treats this as a problem of damp in the body; usually internal damp, caused by an infection or fungus, although it can sometimes be external. Some forms of thrush produce a damp heat, which must be treated with medicine. It is also important to avoid damp food such as sweet or creamy foods. Medicines include Chinese gentian or oriental wormwood.

Thyroid disorders

The thyroid gland lies in the neck at the Adam's apple, immediately in front of the windpipe, and produces the iodine-containing substances that control the rate of metabolism (the pace of chemical activity in all the body cells). It therefore affects mental and physical growth and development. The thyroid is in turn controlled by the pituitary gland at the base of the skull, which secretes thyroid-stimulating hormone.

A goitre is formed by the swelling of the thyroid gland. It can be caused by a lack of iodine in the diet, but it can also be caused by overgrowth, or may be due to a tumour which in very rare cases may be malignant.

An underactive thyroid can develop gradually. It can cause weight gain, and lethargy, and a sufferer will tend to sleep more than usual. The skin and hair become dry and there may be some hair loss. The eyes become puffy and the voice deepens.

An overactive thyroid results in an excess of the thyroid hormones in the blood. This speeds up the metabolic rate, and sufferers lose weight, become restless and fidgety, and find it difficult to sleep. They can suffer from palpitations and sweating, a goitre may develop, and the eyes may bulge.

Overactivity of the thyroid gland is caused by heat in the liver, according to TCM, and can sometimes also be caused by a deficiency in the liver, which may make sufferers hungry, nervous and prone to sweating. The treatment begins by clearing the heat from the liver, in order to restore its balance. Many marine plants and animals are used in the treatment, especially seaweed.

Underactive thyroid glands are usually attributed to spleen deficiency, kidney deficiency and dampness. The treatment will aim to tonify the spleen, tonify the kidneys and remove the dampness inside. Prepared fritillary is often used as a medicine.

Tic

A nervous twitch of a muscle in the face, this is also known as habit spasm. In children, it is often the result of a nervous disposition. Often they are unaware of the tic, and it is best not to call attention to it. In most cases it will disappear of its own accord.

There is no treatment in orthodox medicine, and unless a tic is particularly obvious, and causes embarrassment, it should be forgotten. TCM sees it as a problem of wind in the liver, which can be caused by the heat of the liver or by a liver blood deficiency. Treatment is directed at both the cause of the wind heat or the deficiency, and the symptoms.

Tinnitus

This condition, which causes ringing in the ears, can stem from the ear itself, but may also be caused by high blood pressure and other problems. The source will be rooted in the kidneys. For old people, who are most often affected by tinnitus, the treatment is to tonify the kidneys to strengthen the blood. If the kidney essence is deficient, herbs which can alleviate this include Chinese wolfberry, mulberry fruit and dodder seed. Antelope or deer horn can also be helpful. If the tinnitus is caused by high blood pressure, the treatment would be different. Acupuncture can sometimes be helpful, but for chronic weakness of kidneys, leading to tinnitus, a combination of herbs and acupuncture is best.

Tonsillitis

This can be an extremely painful complaint, causing a very sore throat as the tonsils, which are situated at the back of the throat, become inflamed and swollen. The neck glands are also affected in many cases, and there may be a dry cough. Children get tonsillitis more often than adults, because it is often caused by a virus to which they have not had time to develop resistance. It can also be the result of bacteria.

TCM will diagnose this as due to wind and heat or, sometimes, to fire poison. Heat, poison and fire can be treated internally, for example with honeysuckle flowers drunk as tea. A salt-water gargle can also be used to sterilize locally. The diet can be modified – tonsillitis sufferers should not eat too much spicy food, as that will aggravate the problem. Three-sided acupuncture needles to prick the top of the ears can also be effective.

Toothache

Toothache complicated by some kind of swelling in the gum or elsewhere in the mouth is caused by heat in the stomach. An aching tooth which is not accompanied by swelling is usually caused by a liver problem.

'Stomach' toothache is treated with gypsum to cool the heat or with rhubarb to purge the heat. 'Liver' toothache is best treated with acupuncture, although Chinese ginseng or chrysanthemum flowers can be used as well. For self-help with acute toothache, try a little acupressure. Pressure on the point just in between the thumb and the index finger, held firmly between the thumb and index finger of the opposite hand, can sometimes produce particularly quick results.

Travel sickness

Whether caused by air, sea or land travel, the symptoms of all travel sickness tend to be the same. Acupuncture or acupressure to the stomach points can be useful in combating the feelings of nausea. Medicine such as ginger will be used to warm the stomach.

Ulcerated colitis

Usually treated in two separate ways. Because of the ulceration there is diarrhoea, with mucus and blood in the stool. TCM attributes this to damp, and to heat which burns inside, causes damage to the blood vessels and can become poisoned in the intestine. This poison has to be cleared, and dandelion would be used for this. When the problem is long-term there may also be a spleen deficiency, which will be treated with tonic herbs such as astragalus (see case history, page 54).

Uterine disorders

These include anything from cancer or fibroids to certain kinds of colic or simply infections. TCM is particularly effective against fibroids, especially when sufferers are young and treated early. There are many herbs which can help to dilate and enlarge the uterus, and these can also shrink small fibroids, thus making surgery unnecessary. A good TCM doctor will try to uncover underlying causes to avoid recurrence of fibroids. Herbs used include angelica, rehmannia, sage and remedies such as Women's Precious Pills.

Varicose ulcers

These normally follow varicose veins. In TCM they are connected with stagnation of the blood and qi; this leads to fermenting heat and damp which erupt into ulcers. The damp heat has to be cleared and the circulation of the blood and qi improved. External and internal treatment is given. Corktree bark, peony, rehmannia, angelica and cinnamon twigs clear the damp heat and move the blood. Externally, honey or sesame oil, olive oil or pure sugar can be applied directly on a bandage, which must be kept clean and changed frequently. The sugar draws the damp and the bacteria cannot survive without dampness.

Varicose veins

Bad circulation is a major cause of this common problem, in which the veins become knotted, lengthened and distended. Although the legs are most commonly affected, veins inside the rectum may also become varicose (see Haemorrhoids) and can also occasionally occur around the vulva in pregnancy.

In the case of leg veins, the blood flow becomes obstructed in the rectum and causes the one-way valve on the veins to lose their efficiency, allowing the blood to flow backwards. The result is increased pressure and distension. People who spend long periods standing are particularly susceptible, and it is one of the problems of pregnancy for many women.

Varicose veins can lead to more serious complications, and TCM treatment involves moving the qi and the blood in the body. Chinese angelica, astragalus and cinnamon twigs are commonly used. There are also herbal medicines which can be used externally. Honey can help to sterilize the area where the veins are ulcerated and hasten the regrowth of the skin.

Vertigo

Sufferers feel that their head is spinning when in fact it is quite still. The condition is often triggered by fear of falling from a height, or during bouts of nausea and vomiting. Vertigo can be caused by inflammation of the balance organ in the inner ear, or by some other ear disorder. It is a frequent symptom in cases of high blood pressure.

TCM identifies three possible causes: a deficiency of the blood and the qi (common in old people or after serious illness), or liver wind or phlegm in the body. Each is easily treated with herbs, once the doctor has isolated the cause.

Virus infections

Although the concept of virus infection does not exist in TCM, it does recognize epidemics and is successful in treating both hepatitis and flu. Honeysuckle and oriental wormwood, for example, are good for hepatitis. In addition, recent research into viruses in China has yielded encouraging results. In one study, early results appeared to show that some herbs can kill viruses in the same way as antibiotics can kill bacteria. If confirmed, this could offer great hope for all virus-connected conditions, including AIDS.

Warts

In TCM warts are attributed to the weakness of the liver, which has been invaded by wind heat. Acupuncture treatment is good for this, or a herbal plaster will burn off the wart. Internally, the liver should be cooled and nourished by dandelion, wild chrysanthemum, sage, red peony and oyster shell made into a tea, and drunk regularly. This will ensure that the warts do not return.

Weight problems

The common perception about people who are overweight is that they become that way through overeating, but this is not necessarily the case. Some people eat less than others, yet still put on weight. There are two points of influence here – what you eat and what you are. Some people have a more efficient metabolism than others, and process the food more efficiently. Too many fatty foods and dairy products are not good for the system, particularly in someone with a tendency to gain weight. Rice and vegetables is a much more sensible diet. It may not be necessary to eat less, just to change your eating habits.

People with a sluggish metabolism, it is thought in TCM, produce a lot of internal phlegm and dampness owing to a weakness of the kidneys and spleen. They should eat more 'warm' food. Spleen and kidney tonics may be prescribed by the doctor. Exercise will also help.

People who are underweight may either not be eating enough, or not be eating well enough. Others who eat well yet cannot gain weight need help with their stomach and intestines, to help them absorb food more efficiently. People with diabetes who lose weight are thought to need help with the kidneys. It is not possible to list the herbs that could be used to treat weight problems, as this is very much an individual matter, dependent upon the patient. A TCM doctor will prescribe accordingly.

Appendix:
The Ancient Manuscripts

The Tao gives rise to one,
The one gives rise to two,
The two gives rise to three,
The three produce ten thousand things,
The ten thousand things all
carry yin on their shoulders and
embrace yang in their arms.

Even in the West, the most famous symbol of all things Chinese is the circle of the Tao. Within it, two shapes like tadpoles are interlinked, swimming in opposite directions. The upper tadpole is white with a black 'eye', and the tadpole beneath is black with a white 'eye'.

These are yin and yang, of which all things are made, and which are opposite but indivisible. Each creates and controls the other, each perpetually transforms into the other. Within yang, which is light, rising, exterior, excess and heat, is an element of yin (the black eye). Within yin, which is dark, descending, interior, deficient and cold, is an element of yang (the white eye).

These are the insignia of Taoism, the natural philosophy which prevailed in China long before recorded history, and which remains at the root of Chinese thought, forming the essence of the national character. It evolved through early man's closeness to the earth and acute observation of nature. Tao means 'the Way'. It teaches harmony, moderation, and adherence to the natural law will enhance and prolong life. Like all things Chinese, it is at once the epitome of simplicity, yet of a complexity on a par with Einstein's theory of relativity.

Joseph Needham, the distinguished Sinologist, scientist and historian, in his major work, *Science and Civilization in China*, suggests that the book of the Tao, the *Tao Te Ching*, 'the most profound and beautiful work in the Chinese language', is primarily an explanation of the beginning of the universe. It teaches that when the cosmos was formed through an event in which force, form and substance divided, the lighter and purer substances rose to form heaven, and the heavier and coarser sank to make the earth.

The mystical obscurity of the verse becomes immediately relevant to modern cosmology, if the One is thought of as an electron. The Tao gives rise to an electron. Combined with a proton, it produces an atom. Out of the atom comes the molecule, out of the molecule, comes matter, the 'ten thousand things', an archaic phrase meaning 'everything'.

The *Nei Jing*, the *Yellow Emperor's Classic of Internal Medicine*, explains that 'The principle of Yin and Yang is the basis of the entire universe. It brings about the transformation to parenthood, it is the root and source of life and death . . . Heaven was created by an accumulation of yang, the earth was created by an accumulation of yin.'

When the Chinese talk of qi, they are referring to energy, to matter. Qi exists in different forms. Where there is matter, life is created, through evolution under the right conditions. In nature, the mechanism of polarity is paramount. Everything has its opposite.

Chinese medical theory, from the time of the *Nei Jing*, is based upon the Tao. The human being is both part of the cosmos and has a separate and internal cosmos. To enjoy good health and a long life, people should follow 'the Way'.

The spiritual father of Taoism is Lao Tzu, who was the Keeper of the Archives in Chou State during the fifth or sixth century BC. Although Taoism existed long before this time, he is credited with authorship of the *Tao Te Ching*. As with all the ancient Chinese sages, fact and fantasy are intermingled in his story. Legend tells that he was born with white hair after seventy-two years' gestation and disappeared on a mysterious journey into the sunset mounted on an ox.

The more prosaic version of his life, that he gave up public office to study the Tao and to write his book, is undoubtedly the more reliable. The other details are probably meant to explain that it took a lifetime to attain great wisdom, and that he lived to a great age by following the Tao. His mysterious journey is the one that everybody takes, when life is ended. Little is known of the man behind the myth. His real name is thought to be Li Erh. Lao Tzu is simply a title, meaning Old Master.

Taoism began as a straightforward philosophy, but through the ages became distorted by alchemy, religious mysticism and the occult. The simple message that a long and serene life is the natural consequence of living in harmony with the seasons, without materialistic longings, without hatred or anger, was taken out of context.

Certain schools of Taoists began to search for an elixir which would allow disciples to live forever. At least four rulers are said to have died as the result of drinking various brews which were concocted to achieve this. When the *Nei Jing* was written, however, it acknowledged the Tao in its purest form. It spoke of the 'spiritual beings' who had once lived upon the earth in perfect health for more than 100 years, without any loss of their natural vigour because they 'shunned vain strivings and heedless exertions', and it advocated a similar pattern of behaviour for those who wanted to enjoy a long, healthy and untroubled existence.

The Yellow Emperor, Huang Ti, was himself 'a perfectly accomplished spirit' who was said to have invented the wheel, writing, ships, armour, the nine needles of acupuncture and many other scientific advances. His wife is credited with showing the Chinese how to rear silkworms on mulberry leaves to make silk.

Huang Ti was one of three Celestial Emperors who are said to have lived during a legendary period in history which lasted 647 years between 2852 and 2205 BC. The first, Fu-hsi, was the emperor of heaven. The second, the Red Emperor, Shen Nung, was emperor of earth, the patron of herbalists and apothecaries and author of *The Great Herbal*. He bestowed upon humanity the 'five grains' so that they could avoid killing animals, and taught the human race how to treat illness with medicinal herbs and other substances. Huang Ti, most revered of all, was emperor of mankind. Pictures of the three hang in every TCM medical school and hospital in China: Fu-hsi, grave, scholarly and serene, Shen Nung, fierce with his ox-like head, and his tunic of leaves, and the Yellow Emperor venerable and benign, with his long white beard.

Huang Ti's *Classic of Internal Medicine* remains the most authoritative at source work of TCM. The *Nei Jing* is in two books, the *Su Wen*, or *Plain Questions*, and the *Ling Shu*, sometimes translated as *The Miraculous Pivot*, meaning to pass the gate spiritually or mystically.

Huang Ti recommended dissection as a way of learning anatomy. He weighed the tongue, recorded the twelve pairs of main vessels for the circulation of the blood, noted the arteries, veins and capillaries, the twelve pairs of ligaments, and the 365 acupuncture points. All the theory echoes the theme of the body as a cosmos: twelve for the months of the year, 365 for the days. It explains the functions of the organs as the administration of a state, with the heart as the emperor, the lungs as ministers, the liver as a general, and so on.

Various translations have been disputed and re-interpreted as Chinese medicine advanced, but the *Nei Jing* remains the text which all Chinese doctors study first and last. The book is probably a compilation of accumulated medical lore and wisdom, but its insight into the human body is so comprehensive and sophisticated that some Chinese regard it as, if not divine in origin, then an example of inherent rather than acquired knowledge: medical wisdom which primitive man may have been born with, just as certain species of bird are born with their own internal compass, or some creatures are hatched from the egg and emerge into the world without parents to teach them.

The doctors who wrote books which interpreted the *Nei Jing*, and outlined their own medical findings, were certainly flesh and blood characters, but because TCM has such a long history, even these celebrated physicians are surrounded by myth and legend. In the years that followed the *Nei Jing*, eleven of them became deified and their tablets were worshipped in a special temple, an honour which the physicians themselves would possibly not have approved, being men of science and not superstition.

No one can say for certain when they all lived, or which of the stories attributed to them are true. Some of the most famous medical textbooks no longer exist in their original form. They have either been lost or destroyed, and are only known because of the dissertations or commentaries that later doctors wrote on them. There were regular periods of book burning throughout the ages, and the persecution of scholars seems to have continued as a characteristic of Chinese life right up until the present time. China's First Emperor, who united the seven Warring States into one country ('China' derives from his family name, Chhin), was a military man with a contempt, if not a fear, of intellectuals. He built the Great Wall, and the Warrior Tomb at Xian, but he had 460 scholars condemned to death as an example to others, and decreed that many books should be burned.

Chairman Mao had a similar disdain for intellectuals. When he reorganized the country's medical system (which he did with extreme thoroughness and resounding success) he curtailed the study period by announcing that: 'The more books you read, the more stupid you get.' Medical students in the 1950s were told that their first priority was to get out into the countryside and improve the general health of the people. At the time of China's liberation the population was worn out with warfare and internal strife, ill-nourished and ravaged by disease. Within a few years, a simple but effective health service had been established, and many epidemic diseases were controlled.

Before the Communist revolution, medical students had always followed a tradition of apprenticeship, either to doctors or herbalists, so that they learned by practical experience and inherited the particular prescriptions or the secret formulae of their masters, but they studied the classical texts as well as assisting at consultations. At certain moments in history, when physicians were celebrated as 'the hand of the nation', colleges were established and a strict examination system was set up. At other times, medicine fell back into a disorganized state where even the best doctors were classed alongside any old quack or charlatan who sold charms and spells to treat disease. As we saw in Chapter 2, Confucius and his followers did not regard the study of medicine as a suitable occupation for gentlemen, and Confucianism remained the official philosophy of the state until 1905.

Throughout the ages, however, the common people, whose health and well-being depended on the advance of medical knowledge, always appreciated a skilled practitioner, as did the emperor and his court. Even in state examinations for court officials, applicants were tested on their medical knowledge, since it was thought that a well-rounded student should have a basic understanding of the human body and the nature and treatment of disease, even if his ultimate goal was to be an administrator or a high civil servant. But medical knowledge was appreciated rather than revered.

Some doctors, the famous Hua Tuo among them, always deplored their lowly status on the social ladder. Others were monks and scholars who preferred study and seclusion to the rewards of the material world. They continued to follow the science of medicine because they had a gift for healing and a fascination with research. They enjoyed experiment and clinical observation, and regarded the furtherance of knowledge which could benefit mankind as its own reward.

The celebrated Bian Que, also called Ch'in Yueh-jen, said to be the greatest diagnostician of all time is credited with authorship of the *Nan Jing*, or *Difficult Classic*, which explained some of the more obscure parts of the *Nei Jing*. All down the ages, doctors subjected the growing list of medical textbooks to scrutiny and re-evaluation, correcting misapprehensions as knowledge advanced, and recording their own theories and findings.

The 8,000 classical texts in the treasure-house of Chinese medical literature are valued as important historical documents as well as for their erudition. They trace the development of medicine as a thriving science when the West was still in the dark ages, and when modern science dismisses TCM as unscientific, they offer definitive proof to the contrary. Fortunately the First Emperor of China, Chhin Shih Huang Ti, the self-styled Yellow Emperor, spared most of the medical texts during his book-burning purges.

In the Han Dynasty which followed Chhin's fourteen-year rule, the capital of China remained in Xian, in the north of the country where the climate was harsh and the people suffered the illnesses associated with cold weather. It was at this period, around 176 BC, that Chinese medicine proper begins.

Not surprisingly, the best doctors served the court, and it was this which prompted Zhang Zhong-jing, often called the Chinese Hippocrates, and revered as one of the greatest sages of traditional medicine, to write his famous book the *Shang Han Za Bing Lun*, or *Treatise on Febrile Diseases*. 'Shang Han' is a generic term, meaning ailments caused by external factors, and covers a variety of diseases from a simple chill to gastritis, typhoid or cholera.

Zhang taught that there were six levels of disease which invaded the six pairs of channels, beginning externally and penetrating deeper into the body. He advocated special diets for illness, and gave 113 prescriptions, the first of their kind, most of which are still used today. He also administered enemas and colonic irrigation as part of his treatments. Zhang wrote other famous books, all of which were works of literature with a high moral tone. For him, the practice of medicine was a noble mission to heal the sick and to eliminate the ignorance and credulity of the general public. His writings were edited and preserved by a doctor called Wang Xi (210–85) who also produced a standard work of his own, the *Mai Jing*, or *Pulse Classic*, which systemized and perfected the art of pulse reading.

Two other renowned medical sages practised around the time of Zhang. Hua Tuo, known as 'the God of Surgery' is thought to have been born around AD 190. A long list of his cases is recorded in the Wei and Han Annals, and he is known to have developed an anaesthetic called mafeisan, 'bubbling wine', which may have had an opium or cannabis base. The prescription for this was lost because Hua Tuo incurred a ruler's wrath and was condemned to death.

Doctors led hazardous lives in those days. They were honoured and valued by the emperors as long as they could cure the sick, but the greater their prestige, the more precarious their position. Hua Tuo was kept at court, and realized it was merely a matter of time until he was presented with a case he could not cure. He made the excuse that his mother was ill, and returned home to An Wei province, with no intention of returning. Each time the Emperor requested his return, Hua Tuo employed some new delaying tactic.

When the Emperor realized that he was being defied, he ordered Hua Tuo's arrest and execution. The night before he died, the physician is said to have given all his papers to his gaoler, asking him to hide them until it was safe to pass them on to other doctors. The gaoler was too frightened of what his own fate might be if the papers were discovered, to do what he was asked. He burned them all, and only one page was recovered from the flames. It outlined the surgical procedure for castration, carried out on the eunuchs who served the females of the Emperor's household.

This practice continued until the turn of the last century, and barbaric though it sounds, it was a passport to a life of comparative luxury and ease for those who were prepared to pay the price of mutilation. Applicants traditionally came from the village of Hochienfu, a city 100 miles south of Tianjin. Operators known as 'knifers' kept the trade in their own families and worked from a special establishment at the gates of the palace.

First they bathed the penis and scrotum in a hot decoction of peppers. The applicant, if an adult, was then asked three times if he repented, or ever would repent, his decision. Most went ahead with the operation, and while they were held down, all the parts were swept away in one stroke of a special sickle-shaped knife. A pewter plug was then inserted into the urethra, and the patient, supported by two men, was walked up and down for three hours. For the next three days they were given nothing to drink, and at the end of that period the plug was removed, and the dressings changed. Healing took 100 days, and only 2 per cent of the operations proved fatal.

Hua Tuo invented sutures, performed abdominal operations, and was the first to use antiseptics and anti-inflammatory ointments. He promoted the idea of hydrotherapy – still widely used in Chinese hospitals – and was an expert in acupuncture and moxibustion techniques, devising a way for doctors to find the right acupoints in each patient, regardless of their height or girth, by measuring certain parts of the body and using them as 'units' to gauge the precise locations. A series of acupoints are named after him.

Hua Tuo was said to use few drugs, but was so accurate in dispensing that he did not bother to weigh the ingredients. His operations were so successful, it is said, that a wound sutured by him would be cleared in five days and cured within a month. Yet surgery continued to have a lowly status, and its development remained impeded, because of the religious stigma that attached to it.

Despite the fact that at certain times in Chinese history surgery and dissection were not only practised but officially encouraged, the predominant attitude was always very ambivalent. Confucius had instilled in the nation an idea of the sanctity of the body as a gift from the ancestors, and this tenet persisted regardless of recorded surgical techniques, one of which included correcting a hare lip.

Another eminent physician of the time was Chun Yu-i, a dedicated clinician who kept detailed case histories in order to check the effectiveness of treatments. His abrupt manner brought him into disfavour at court, and he too was sentenced to death, possibly on a trumped-up charge. When he learned his fate, Chun bemoaned the fact that he had no son to defend his name, and the youngest of his five daughters, on hearing this, set out to ask the Emperor to spare her father's life.

The ruler demanded proof of Chun's skills as a doctor, and his clinical records were sent to court, where they so impressed that the physician's life was spared. His fame has been handed down through the centuries in anecdotal form. He emphasized the importance of pulse-reading, and was said to have treated cancer, cystitis, rheumatism, paralysis and kidney disease. He brought a scientific detachment to his practice, and freely admitted his mistakes, but he left no written works.

A celebrated book intended 'to cut out inconsistencies and repetitions' from the *Nei Jing* was written by a literary scholar called Huangfu-Mi. He started life as a historian and a poet, but was led to medicine because of his mother's paralysis, and because he himself suffered from severe rheumatism. His book, A *Classic of Acupuncture and Moxibustion*, is a comprehensive work outlining the names and numbers of all the acupoints, explaining the depth at which the needles should be inserted, and the length of time they should stay in place. He detailed the method of needling to tonify and sedate, and his book remains a standard reference work which is still relevant to acupuncturists today.

Some of the later Taoists also studied medicine. One of the most famous alchemists, Ge Hong, or Bao Puzi, as he is sometimes called, was a doctor as well. He came from a poor family and had to work as a labourer to pay for his education, which may be why his overriding concern was to bring good, reliable and inexpensive medicines within reach of the common people. Two of his books, *Prescriptions from the Golden Box* and *A Handbook of Prescriptions for Emergencies*, are dedicated to that end.

Some of his prescriptions were later discovered carved in Buddhist caves at the Dragon's Gate in Tun Huang, together with medical remedies advocated by another master Taoist whose work he greatly influenced. Tao Hong Jing was one of those exceptionally gifted people who excel at many subjects. He was an astronomer, calligrapher, mathematician and pharmacologist. He was influenced as much by Buddhism as Taoism, and gave up life as a court official to live as a hermit in the mountains. There he wrote a commentary on Shen Nung's *Great Herbal*, which became one of the most valuable books of Materia Medica in China.

Life cloistered from the world seemed to be the safest location for pioneering doctors, but still their fame reached the capital. Sun Si-Miao, who lived during the Tang Dynasty, began a life of learning and contemplation at the age of seven, and withdrew to the Tapo mountains to live as a hermit, devoting his life to the study of herbs. He wrote two of the most famous of the medical classics, *Prescriptions Worth a Thousand Gold Pieces* and a second volume which was a supplement to the first.

Among his many pioneering treatments was to prescribe goat or rabbit liver for patients suffering from night blindness. This is now recognized to be the result of deficiency of Vitamin A, in which liver is rich. Under Sun's direction, a hospital was set up for lepers. Two emperors tried to lure him to court with offers of high position, but he wisely declined, pleading ill-health, and stayed at the hermitage. He died at the age of 101.

Doctors followed who specialized in paediatrics, forensic medicine and gynaecology, and various other areas. The first book on paediatrics was published in AD 1119. It recorded the work of Qian Yi, a court physician who had over forty years of experience treating children, and probably began his career around the time of the Norman Conquest in Britain. He was the first to point out the particular features of paediatric medicine, and advanced new theories of diagnosis and treatment which had a profound influence on its development. The book, *Key to the Therapeutics of Children's Diseases*, was actually compiled by his student Yan Xiao-zhong.

The concept that stress could cause illness was first proposed in the twelfth century by Chen Yan, in the theory of three causes, suggesting that all disease sprang either from endogenous factors such as sorrow, distress or fear, or exogenous caused by climatic conditions, or by random happenings and mischance, like snake bite, a wound or an accident.

During this period, several schools of thought evolved, attributing disease to different factors, each advocating contrasting approaches to treatment. Zhang Cong-zheng was a court physician who regarded disease as a foreign substance in the organism which should be driven out by diaphoretics, emetics or purgatives. Around the same time, Li Gao founded the School for Strengthening Spleen and Stomach, teaching that illness mainly stemmed from internal injury caused by intemperance and overwork.

Zhu Zhen-heng, the Master of Danxi, believed that indulgence was the root of all illness with yang usually in excess, and yin often deficient. He was founder of the School for Nourishing the Yin by means oftonic herbs, and his two classics, On Inquiring into the *Properties of Things and Expounding the Formulating of the Bureau of the People's Welfare Pharmacies,* were published around 1350.

Dietary rules for the promotion of good health and the treatment of sickness were laid down in the masterwork of a Mongolian chef in the imperial household during the Yuan

Dynasty. Hu Si-hui wrote *Principles of Correct Diet* in 1330. Even today, the Chinese firmly hold to the view that food is also a medicine, and they eat accordingly. If they could also be persuaded that cigarettes are a poison, they might avoid the inevitable consequence of heart disease, cancers and strokes which they now suffer from as much as people in the Western world. In mainland China, smoking is so commonplace and so popular that guests are offered a cigarette not just between courses, but actually *with* food. In restaurants in many of the large cities, a quick inhalation of nicotine is regarded as the perfect accompaniment to soup.

It is a strange aberration in a country otherwise so well informed about health care and self-diagnosis, and although the government does make some effort to conduct campaigns warning about the effects of smoking, nobody seems to take much notice. The chainsmoking boss of a large pharmaceutical factory advocated cigarettes as an answer to stress. They were very good for calming the nerves, he said. It can be argued that all forms of deep breathing have this effect, and in practices like qi gong, only air is taken into the system. Anyone wishing to see the effect of cigarette-smoking on a vast country like China has only to look at the mortality statistics. A School on the True Understanding of Nicotine is long overdue.

It was concern about toxins which inspired one of China's greatest scientists in his lifetime's work. During the Ming Dynasty in 1518, a boy was born in Hubei province who proved to be rather a disappointment to his family. Several generations had produced doctors, but Li Shi zhen preferred to become a court official. After failing his county examinations three times, however, he decided to try medicine after all, and at twenty-three years of age set out on a ten-year course of study.

He realized that the existing pharmaceutical works had no consistent classification, and contained mistakes, duplications and omissions. Worse, they also listed poisons from the heyday of the alchemists, in their bizarre search for immortality. Many people had died through taking these concoctions, and it was 400 years since the last pharmacopeia had been published. Despite the advances of medical knowledge during those centuries, the herbal listings had never been properly updated.

For the next thirty years, Li dedicated himself to the study of medicinal plants. He travelled far and wide, visiting famous medical scholars, researching and investigating old remedies, and going out over the mountains and the steppes on plant-hunting expeditions. His *Outline of Materia Medica* runs to fifty-two volumes, providing the most comprehensive information about the taste, action, dosage and side-effects of herbs.

Li also listed waters, soils, gems, vegetables, fruits, trees, insects, fish, poultry and animals, and discussed the aetiology and treatment of 100 diseases. The work, written between 1552 and 1578, is internationally celebrated as one of the world's great monuments of scholarship. Li also wrote a book on the pulse, and another, *The Eight Extra Channels*, which greatly advanced the science of acupuncture.

It was during the Ming Dynasty that Wu Youxing developed his theory of 'foul and evil, foreboding air' causing epidemics. The idea that contagion could be breathed in through the nose or mouth was a departure from the old idea that disease penetrated the body from its surface. Medicine flourished at this time, with specialist works on eye disease, paediatrics, syphilis.

When the Ming empire fell, one of its gifted officials went into hiding to fight against the ruling Qing. Fu Quin-zhu was a poet, painter and calligrapher as well as a physician. His many medical books could not be printed under his own name at the time they were written, and it was not until last century, some 200 years after his death, that extracts from them were published again and the author identified in *Fu Qing-zhu's Obstetrics and Gynaecology* and *Fu Quin-zhu's Work on Women's Diseases*.

Once the influence of the West began to pervade mainland China, traditional medicine was destined to decline in popularity, but doctors still continued to further their knowledge. Vaccination, and its increasing use in China, was one of the main topics by a distinguished medical author, Zhang-Lu, who wrote a sixteen-volume treatise, *On Medicine*. He was born in 1617, and the work took him fifty years to complete.

A famous physician of the Qing Dynasty, Wang Ang, established that the brain was the source of mental activities and memory, and not the heart, as had previously been thought. He was very broadminded about the advent of Western medicine, which was just beginning to get a foothold in China, but unfortunately it was to herald a decline in the fortunes of TCM, which would last until the mid-twentieth century.

Mao Zedong set up academies of Chinese medicine in all the country's major cities in 1949. The task of preparing standard editions of all the existing literature on Chinese medicine was begun in 1954. Four years later, the two systems were formally given equal status, and in January 1986, the State Council of the People's Republic set up the State Administration Bureau of TCM and Pharmacy.

Even today, in an integrated system, TCM gets the lesser share of the nation's resources, but as it advances in the West, offering treatments such as acupuncture which can treat conditions like intractable pain at a fraction of the cost of expensive long-term drug therapies, and herbal medicines which are far more effective at treating chronic conditions than many modern synthetic remedies, TCM is almost certainly on the verge of a new renaissance. Perhaps in the not far distant future, TCM and conventional medicine will begin to merge in the West, absorbing the best of both systems into a new framework offering the whole of humanity new hope in conquering suffering and disease.

Useful Addresses

Further Information

For further advice on treatment and courses on Traditional Chinese Medicine, Dr Ke can be contacted at the Asante Academy of Chinese Medicine in London, UK. (http://www.asante-academy.com)

Professor Song Ke (MB MBAcC FRCHM MATCM FRSM)

The Asanté Academy of Chinese Medicine, Clerkenwell Building, Archway Campus, 2-10 Highgate Hill, London, N19 5LW. Tel: +44 (0) 20 7272 6888. Fax: +44 (0) 20 7272 1998 info@asante-academy.com

TCM schools

Pui-Yong Post Graduate School of TCM, 53a Ormistone Grove, London W12 0JP. Tel: 0181 743 0706. Students must be scientists or health professionals with qualifications equivalent to BSc.

Fook Sang Acupuncture and Chinese Herbal Practitioners Association. HQ: 590 Wokingham Road, Earley, Reading, Berks RG6 2HN. Tel: 01734 665454. Prefers entrants with Western medicine qualifications, but will under some circumstances take students with no medical background. Three-year study course.

College of Oriental Medicine, Prospect House, Retford, Nottinghamshire DN22 6NA. Tel: 01777 701509. Variety of courses in medicine and acupuncture from four-day programmes for health professionals to intensive two-year programmes in Chinese acupuncture and moxibustion.

The International College of Oriental Medicine, Green Hedges Avenue, East Grinstead, Sussex RH19 1DZ. Tel: 01342 313106.

School of Chinese Herbal Medicine, Midsummer Cottage Clinic, Nether Westcote, Kingham, Oxon. OX7 6SD. Tel: 01993 830419. (The school is based in central London.)

Associations

The Association of Traditional Chinese Medicine, 78 Haverstock Hill, London NW3 2BE. Tel: 0171 284 2898.

The Register of Chinese Herbal Medicine, 2 Warbeck Road, London W12 8NS.

Qigong

LONDON

The British Qigong College, 2 St Albans Road, London NW5 1RD.
Simon Lau, Eastern Horizon Studio, 28 Old Brompton Road, South Kensington, London SW7 3DL.

Bruce Kumar Frantzis, c/o Brian Cooper, 85m Davey Drive, Brighton BN1 7BJ.

Kalil Quin, 2 West Heath Drive, London NW11.

Master Lam Kam Chuen, The Lam Clinic, 70 Shaftesbury Avenue, London W1V 7DF

BRISTOL

Mark Caldwell, The Healing Tao Foundation, 3 Redcliffe Parade East, Bristol BS1 6SW.

Ross, Greenfields Qigong Centre, 2 Rockleaze Ave, Sneyd Park, Bristol BS9 1NG.

Bill Harpe, The Blackie, Great Georges Community Cultural Project, Great George Street, Liverpool L1 5EW.

MANCHESTER

Linda Chase Broda, The Village Hall, 163 Palatine Road, Manchester M20 8GH.

Danny Connor, The Qigong Institute, 18 Swan Street, Manchester, M4 5JN.

Michael Tse, Tse Qigong Centre, PO Box 116, South D.O., Manchester M20 9YN.

NEWCASTLE ON TYNE

Bi Song Guo, 12 Church Lane, Gosforth, Newcastle on Tyne.

Sifu Peter Young, PE International, 176 Helmsley Road, Newcastle on Tyne NE2 1RD.

READING

John and Angela Hicks, The College of Integrated Chinese Medicine, 40 College Road, Reading, Berkshire RG6 1QB.

RUGBY

John Harford, Nei Chia, The Farmhouse, Corner Farm, Ashby St Ledgers, Rugby, Warwickshire CV23 8UN.

SCOTLAND

Larry Butler, 5 West Bank Quadrant, Glasgow G12 8AF.

WALES

Richard Farmer, Rising Dragon School, The White House, Maryland, Nr Trellech, Monmouth, Gwent NP5 4QJ.

Acupuncture

British Medical Acupuncture Society, Newton House, Newton Lane, Lower Whitley, Warrington, Cheshire WA4 4JA. Tel: 01925 730727.

British Acupuncture Association & Register, 34 Alderney Street, London SW1V 4EU. Tel: 0171 834 1012

Chung San Acupuncture Society, 15 Porchester Gardens, London W2 4DB.

International Register of Oriental Medicine UK. 4 The Manor House, Colley Lane, Reigate, Surrey RH2 9JW. Tel: 0171 727 6778.

Traditional Acupuncture Society, 1 The Ridgeway, Stratford-upon-Avon, Warwickshire CV37 9JL. Tel: 01789 298798.

Register of Traditional Chinese Medicine, 19 Trinity Road, London N2 8JJ. Tel: 0181 883 8431.

Association of British Veterinary Acupuncture, East Park Cottage, Handcross, Haywards Heath, Sussex RH1 6BD. Tel: 01342 400213.

Self-help and support groups

Action Against Allergy, 24/26 High Street, Hampton Hill, Mddx TW12 1PD.

A1 Anon Family Groups, UK & Eire (support for families of alcoholics), Box 514, 11 Redcliffe Gardens, London SW10 9BQ. Tel: 0171 833 3471.

Alcoholics Anonymous, PO Box 514, 11 Redcliffe Gardens, London SW10 9BQ. Tel: 0171 833 3471.
Alzheimer's Disease Society, Gordon House, 10 Greencoat Place, London SW1P 1PH. Tel: 0171 3060606.

Alzheimer's Scotland, 8 Hill Street, Edinburgh EH2 3JZ. Tel: 0131 225 1453.

Arthritis Care, 18 Stephenson Way, London NW1 2HD. Tel: 0171 916 1500 (also advises about Lupus).

Back Pain Association, 16 Elmstree Road, Teddington, Middx, TW1 1ST. Tel: 0181 977 5474.

British Association of Cancer United Patients (BACUP), 3 Bath Place, Rivington Street, EC2A 3JR. Tel: 0800 181199.

British Diabetic Association, 10 Queen Anne Street, London W1M 0BD. Tel: 0171 323 1531.

British Epilepsy Association, Anstay House, 40 Hanover Square, Leeds LS3 1BE. Tel: 01132 089599.

British Migraine Association, 178A High Road, Byfleet, West Byfleet, Surrey KT14 7ED. Tel: 01932 352 468.

British Tinnitus Association, c/o Royal National Institute for the Deaf, 105 Gower Street, London WC1E 6AH. Tel: 0171 387 8033.

Cancer Link, 17 Britannia Street, London WC1X 9JN. Tel: 0171 833 2451. 9 Castle Terrace, Edinburgh EH1 2DP. Tel: 0131 228 5557.

Chest, Heart and Stroke Association, CHSA House, Whitecross Street, London EC1Y 8JJ. Tel: 0171 490 7999.

Council for Complementary and Alternative Medicine, 179 Gloucester Place, London NW1 6DX. Tel: 0171 724 9103.

Cystic Fibrosis Trust, Alexandra House, 5 Blyth Road, Bromley, Kent BR1 3RS. Tel: 0181 464 7211.

Disabled Living Foundation, 380-384 Harrow Road, London W9 2HU. Tel: 0171 289 6111.

Drinkline, 13-14 West Smithfield, London EC1A 9DH. Tel: 0171 332 0150. (Information and advice to callers worried about their own drinking. Support to family and friends.)

Eating Disorders Association, Sackville Place, 44 Magdalen Street, Norwich, Norfolk 1JU. Tel: 01603 621 414.

Enuresis Resource and Information Centre, 65 St Michael's Hill, Bristol BS2 8DZ. Tel: 01179 264 920.

Endometriosis Society, 65 Holmdene Ave, Herne Hill, London SE24 9LD. Tel: 0171 737 4764.

Epilepsy Association of Scotland, 48 Govan Road, Glasgow G51 1JL. Tel: 0141 427 4911.

Family Heart Association, 7 High Street, Kidlington, Oxon OX5 2DH. Tel: 01865 370 292. (For families with an inherited risk of coronary heart disease.)

Guillain Barre Syndrome Support Group, Foxley, Holdingham, Sleaford, Lincs. NG34 8NR. Tel: 01529 304615.

Hodgkin's Disease Association, PO Box 275, Haddenham, Aylesbury, Bucks HP17 8JJ. Tel: 01844 291 500.

Intractable Pain Society of Great Britain and Ireland, Pain Relief Clinic, Basingstoke District Hospital, Aldermaston Road, Basingstoke, Hants, RG24 9NA. Tel: 01256 473202.

Issue (National Fertility Association) 509 Aldridge Road, Great Barr, Birmingham. Tel: 0121 344 4414.

Lupus UK, 51 North Street, Romford, Essex RM1 1BA. Tel: 01708 731 251.

ME Association, Stanhope House, High Street, Stanford-Le-Hope, Essex SS17 0HA. Tel: 01375 361 013.

MIND, Granta House, 15-19 Broadway, Stratford, London E15 4BQ. Tel: 0181 519 2122.
Miscarriage Association (acknowledging pregnancy loss), Head Office, c/o Clayton Hospital, Northgate, Wakefield, West Yorkshire WF1 3JS. Tel: 01924 200799.

Mobility Information Service, National Mobility Centre, Unit 2A, Atcham Estate, Shrewsbury SY4 4UG. Tel: 01743 761 889. (Advice to the disabled and information packs to drivers and passengers.)

Motor Neurone Disease Association, David Niven House, 10-15 Notre Dame Mews, 61 Derngate, Northampton, NN1 2BG. Tel: 01604 250505.

Muscular Dystrophy Group of Great Britain and Northern Ireland. Prescott House, Prescott Place, London SW4 2BS. Tel: 0171 720 8055.

Multiple Sclerosis Society of Great Britain and Northern Ireland. 25 Effie Road, Fulham, London SW6 1EE. Tel: 0171 736 6267. Helpline: 0171 371 8000.
Scottish Office: 2A North Charlotte Street, Edinburgh EH2 4HR. Tel: 031 225 3600.
Northern Ireland: 34 Annadale Avenue, Belfast BT7 3JJ Tel: 0232 644914.

National Aids Helpline, PO Box 400, London WC2B 6JG. Helpline: 01800 567 123.

National Ankylosing Spondylitis Society, 5 Grosvenor Crescent, London SW1X 7ER. Tel: 0171 235 9585.

National Asthma Campaign, Providence House, Providence Place, London N1 0NT. Tel: 0171 226 2260.

National Association for Colitis and Crohn's Disease (NACC) 98a London Road, St Albans, Herts AL1 1NX.

National Eczema Society, 4 Tavistock Place, London WC1H 9RA. Tel: 0171 388 4097.

National Kidney Federation, 6 Stanley Street, Worksop, Notts S81 7HX. Tel: 01909 487795.

National Meningitis Trust, Fern House, Bath Road, Stroud, Glos GL5 3TJ. Tel: 01453 755049.

Parkinson's Disease Society of the UK, 22 Upper Woburn Place, London WC1H 0RA. Tel: 0171 383 3513.
Positively Women, 5 Sebastian Street, London EC1V 0HE. Tel: 0171 590 5515. (Support service for women with HIV or Aids.)

Psoriasis Association, 7 Milton Street, Northampton, NN2 7JG. Tel: 01604 711129.

Raynaud's and Scleroderma Assocation, 112 Crew Road, Alsager, Cheshire ST7 2JA. Tel: 01270 872776.

Saneline, 199-205 Old Marylebone Road, London NW1 5QP. Tel: 0171 724 8000.

Stroke Association, CHSA House, Whitecross Street, London EC1Y 8JJ. Helpline: 0171 490 7999.

Terrence Higgins Trust, 52–54 Gray's Inn Road, London WC1X 8JU. Tel: 0171 831 0330.

Animal Products and Endangered Species

In China, every town and village has its own folk medicine market, full of products which would strike the Westerner as strictly for the use of wizards and warlocks, and some which we would regard with outright horror and repugnance. Dried snakes and lizards, sea-horses, the gallstones of cows and horses, turtle shells, antelope horns and animal skins will be found among sacks of roots and grasses, tree bark, twigs and blossoms and an assortment of seaweeds and other marine plants. Even bat droppings, dinosaur fossil bones and the scrapings from the bottom of the interior of a wooden stove may be used in mainland folk medicines.

Thankfully, some medicines made from endangered animal species are now being outlawed in China, if a little late in the day. Only in 1993 were rhinoceros horn and tiger bone banned by the Chinese government, in response to powerful pressure from the international community. But the poaching of endangered species continues unabated, and countries like Taiwan, South Korea, Singapore and Hong Kong, are markets for international smugglers. The illegal trade is almost as profitable as trafficking in heroin or cocaine, and the price per gram can sometimes surpass the cost of gold.

Despite the persistent myth that rhinoceros horn is an effective aphrodisiac and cure for impotence, it was actually prescribed for a variety of illnesses and does in fact have components which are used in medicine, including keratin, calcium carbonate and calcium phosphate. It was used as a heat-clearing and blood-cooling drug, and in the treatment of high fever, spasm and convulsion. Bear bile has been shown, in Western medical tests, to be effective in dissolving gallstones. Tiger bone was regarded as one of the most reliable pain relievers in the treatment of rheumatism.

However repugnant the outside world finds the exploitation of endangered creatures, and the horrific poaching trade which supplies it, it has to be remembered that some of these ingredients were brought into use thousands of years ago, when there was still a balance between man and the animal kingdom; before we had the technology for wholesale slaughter; and that China has been a closed community for decades, sometimes unaware and usually largely indifferent to the cares and concerns of the world beyond.

Official attitudes are changing, albeit slowly, and now the government is imposing strict controls on the collection and sale of herbs, banning the use of some species and overseeing and restricting the collection of plants from ecologically sensitive areas.

Sadly, the world's flora is under equal threat, and many rare and irreplaceable botanical specimens are disappearing from our planet due to development and exploitation. In China, some rare herbs may vanish entirely in the development of vast areas of hitherto unspoiled land, and some of the 50,000-plus species contained in the

Chinese Materia Medica, may be lost forever, before scientists can evaluate their properties.

Together with their international colleagues, Chinese scientists are constantly researching many threatened species, and making new discoveries about the effects of some of the active ingredients they contain, but it is a race against time, and not one which they are certain to win.

There remain practices totally abhorrent to the Western world – the cruel process of 'milking' living bears for the bile from their gallbladders is one which animal agencies are attempting to persuade the Chinese to end, so far without success, however. The Chinese government gives official backing to the forty or more 'bear farms' where Asiatic moon bears are imprisoned in cages so small that they cannot stretch or lift their heads. Metal taps are surgically implanted so that their gallbladders can be 'milked' twice weekly – an agonizing and inhumane practice which is a stain on the honour and reputation of a country and a people that have done so much to advance civilization.

Constant pressure from the outside world may eventually bring about a change in attitude, and those interested in doing what they can to bring about change may find it useful to contact some of the animal protection agencies directly involved. These include:

International Fund for Animal Welfare, 12 Springfield House, West Street, Bristol, BS38 7BD.

Environmental Investigation Agency.

Traffic (Trade Records Analysis of Flora and Fauna in Commerce), the world's largest wildlife trade monitoring group co-funded by the World Wildlife Fund.

Convention on International Trade in Endangered Species of Wild Fauna and Flora (Cites).

Caretakers of the Environments International (CEVNO), Nassau-plein 8, 1815 GM, Alkmaar, Netherlands.

Bibliography

Basic Theory of Traditional Chinese Medicine, Shanghai College of TCM Press, 1990

Chi Kung: Cultivating Personal Energy, by James MacRitchie, Element Books, 1994

Chinese Materia Medica, Shanghai College of TCM Press, 1990

Chinese Medical Herbs, by Li-Shi Zhen, Georgetown Press, 1973

Chinese Medicine, by M. Porkert & C. Ullman, Morrow, 1988

Diagnostics of Traditional Chinese Medicine, Shanghai College of TCM Press, 1990

Essential Book of Traditional Chinese Medicine (2 vols.), by Liu Yanchi, Columbia University Press, 1988

Family Guide to Alternative Medicine, Reader's Digest, 1991

Highly Efficacious Chinese Patent Medicines, Shanghai College of TCM Press, 1990

History of Chinese Medicine, by D. & M.J. Hoizey, Edinburgh University Press, 1994

Serve the People, by V. & R. Sidel, Beacon Press, 1973

The Way of Energy, by Lam Kam Chuen, Gaia Books, 1991

The Yellow Emperor's Classic of Internal Medicine, University of California Press, 1966

Index

Abscess 47, 104, 132
Abdominal pains 150, 177
Abortion 79
Abutilon seeds 91
Acanthopanax bark 91, 138, 166
Achyranthes root 86, 89, 93, 166
Acid stomach 132
Acne 116, 132
Aconite 13, 35, 88, 136, 142, 145, 175
Acupressure 118, 150, 156, 163, 166, 170
Acupuncture 21, 22, 23, 24, 108, 116, 117, 118, 124, 136, 137, 138, 139, 140, 141, 143, 150, 152, 153, 155, 156, 158, 163, 165, 166, 168, 170, 171, 172, 173, 174, 175, 177, 178, 179, 180, 182, 183, 190, 191, 193
Acute lymphoblastic leukaemia 165
Addison's disease 187
Adenophora root 87
Adrenal gland 44, 119, 124
Adsuki bean 91
Agastache 87, 92, 93, 94
Agrimonia bud 88
Agrimony 89
AIDS 15, 76, 79, 133
Air-potato yam 88
Akebia 153
Albizia bark 89
Albizia flower 89
Alchemists 109
Alcohol 97, 102, 134
Alismatis rhizome 91
Aloes 87
Amber 85
American ginseng 156
Amnesia 134
Amoebic dysentery 147
Amomum fruit 62, 87, 90, 93, 94, 128, 149
Anaemia 38, 85, 129, 130, 134
Anemarrhenia rhizome 86, 92, 93, 94
Anemone 147
Angelica 154
Angelica pills 177

Angina pectoris 77, 135, 15, 56
Ankylosis spondylitis 52
Anorexia 44, 128, 135
Antelope horn 127, 162, 190
Antibiotics 54, 132, 139, 145, 165, 174
Anus 151, 153
Anxiety 116, 136, 155, 157, 177
Appendicitis 43
Arborvitae seed 89, 92, 93, 95
Arctium fruit 86, 128
Areca peel 91
Areca seed 88, 94, 95
Argyi leaf 88 92, 93
Arisaema tuber 87
Aristolochia fruit 87
Aristolochia stem 91, 92
Arnebia 87
Artemisia 76, 117, 167, 172
Artemisia capillaris Thunberg 76
Arteriosclerosis 137
Arthritis 70, 116, 128, 131, 136, 153, 164
Artificial cow-bezoar 131
Ash bark 87
Asian dandelion 86
Asparagus root 90, 177
Aster root 87
Asthma 12, 36, 37, 54, 68, 77, 85, 87, 116, 117, 122, 128, 137
Astragalus membranaceus 15, 38, 62, 77, 78, 133, 139, 141, 144, 145, 146, 149, 156, 157, 165, 169
Astragalus root 90, 92, 93, 128
Aster 84
Atherton, Dr David 74
Atopy 154
Atractylodes rhizome 87, 93, 94,128
Aucklandia root 88, 93, 94, 95
AZT 76,

Back pain 38, 59, 111, 112, 116, 121, 128, 138
Bad breath 138
Baldness 138
Balloonflower root 140
Bamboo juice 149
Bamboo leaves 139, 144, 153, 174, 179
Bamboo shavings 87, 149

Bao Puzi 200
Barbat skullcap 86
Basil 150
Bath Chinese Medical Centre 147
Batholin cyst 125
Ba Zhen Wan 130
Beancurd 99
Beansprouts 99
Bed-wetting 38, 104, 148
Beef 99
Bell's Palsy 116, 138
Ben Cao 82
Ben Cao Gang Mu 78
Berberis root 86
Betel nut 187
Bian Que 20, 21, 22, 24, 41, 198
Bilirubin 164
Biota tops 88
Bird's nest soup 98
Bistort rhizome 86
Bitter almond 92, 95, 137, 145
Bitter apricot kernel 87
Bitter cardamom 90, 93
Bitter orange 88
Black aconite 13, 155
Blackberry leaves 142
Blackberry lily rhizome 86, 165
Black ginger seed 145, 148, 150, 168
Black plum 90, 92, 93, 95, 157
Bladder 30, 32, 33, 37, 42, 43, 45, 50, 65, 68, 94, 121, 122, 131, 140
Bleeding 88
Blindness 152
Blisters 142, 151
Blood 29, 30, 139, 152, 153, 155, 157, 160, 162, 164, 165, 170, 177, 180
Blood cells 110, 139, 164
Blood deficiency 125, 141, 168, 170
Blood pressure 112, 116, 130, 139, 146, 174, 179
Blurred vision 122, 151
Boat sterculia seed 87
Body fluids 90
Boehmeria root 89
Boils 85, 98
Bone marrow 15, 110, 114, 119
Borneol 89

Bowels 38, 70, 120, 121, 132,144, 145, 146, 153, 172, 185
Brain 17, 23, 38, 110, 119, 134, 145, 148, 167, 168, 169, 170, 177, 185
Brain damage 149, 168, 169
Breathlessness 122
Bright's disease 139
Bronchial disorders 77, 137
Bronchitis 36, 116, 128, 139
Broom 85
Broom cypress fruit 91, 164
Brucea fruit 86
Bruises 131, 188
Bugleweed 89
Bulimia 140
Bupleurum root 86, 93, 94
Burnet root 88
Burns 104, 131
Burred tuber 88, 167
Bursitis 116
Bushcherry seed 87, 93, 95
Buxue Ningshen Pian 130
Bu Zhong Yi Qi Wan 131

Cabbage 101, 124
Cablin patchouli 87
Calabash gourd 91
Calcium 170, 176, 179, 211
Cancer 14, 15, 62, 72, 76, 77, 78, 112, 123, 141, 156, 165
Candida 141, 189
Cape jasmine fruit 86, 92, 95
Carbuncles 85
Cardiovascular complaints 77
Carp 103
Carpesium fruit 88
Carrot 98, 101
Carthamus tinctorius 77
Cassia bark 88
Cassia twigs 90
Cataracts 122, 130, 142
Catarrh 103, 142
Cat-tail pollen 88, 89, 93, 95
Cauldrons 118
Centipeda herb 86
Central nervous system 124, 157, 172
Central Qi Pills 169, 180

Cephalotaxus harringtonia 78
Cerebral palsy 116
Cerebral thrombosis 16
Cervical cancer 123
Cervix 123
Changzheng Hospital 56, 83
Chaenomeles fruit 91
Chamaedaphne leaf and flower 91
Chang Tao-Ling 109
Channels 91, 117
Chaste-tree fruit 86
Chebula fruit 90
Cheese 101
Chemotherapy 138, 141, 156, 165
Chen Yan 201
Cherokee rosehip 90, 130
Chest 120, 122
Chicken 34, 99, 101, 130, 132
Chicken gizzard 140, 148, 158
Chickenpox 142, 183
Chilblains 34, 119, 142
Childbirth 102, 143
Chilli 102
Chinaberry bark 88
Chinese Academy of Medical Sciences 78
Chinese angelica 37, 38, 62, 70, 90, 92, 93, 99, 130, 136, 137, 139, 141, 146, 147, 155, 156, 164, 170, 180
Chinese black bait 185
Chinese blistering beetle 85
Chinese date 90, 154, 170
Chinese ephedra 90
Chinese gall 90
Chinese gentian 167, 170, 189
Chinese gentian grass 155
Chinese golden thread 132, 138, 157, 178, 181,185, 187
Chinese olive 86
Chinese senegar root 149
Chinese snake gourd 76, 79, 133
Chinese star jasmine 91
Chinese wax gourd peel 91
Chinese yam 90, 93, 141, 146, 165, 187
Chlamydia 162
Cholesterol 135

Chrysanthemum flower 86, 92, 93, 139, 142, 144, 145, 149, 152, 154, 163, 178, 179, 182, 191
Chuan Bei Bi Pa Lu 129
Chuang Tzu 109
Chuanxiong rhizome 89, 92, 94, 95
Chun Yu-i 200
Churchill Hospital, London 137
Cibot rhizome 38, 157, 166, 176
Cimicifuga rhizome 86, 180
Cinnabar 85, 89, 182
Cinnamon bark 88, 92, 93, 169, 180
Cinnamon twigs 35, 86, 92, 135, 136, 139, 142, 146, 150, 154, 155, 163, 176
Circulation problems 29, 34, 35, 89, 172
Cirrhosis 155, 165
Clematis root 91
Cloves 88
Codonopsis 90, 146, 175
Coix seed 91
Colds 116, 117, 128
Colic 77, 97, 103, 143
Colitis 54, 55, 116, 129, 143
Colon 143, 164
Coltsfoot 84, 87
Coma 169
Common clubmoss 91
Common day flower 89
Common knot grass 91
Compendium of Materia Medica 202
Conception vessel 117, 118, 121, 122
Confucius 26, 96, 197, 200
Conjunctivitis 119, 125, 144
Constipation 84, 103, 104, 116, 120, 129, 130, 135, 144, 164, 179
Contraceptives 159
Convulsions 169, 183
Coptis root 86, 92, 94, 95
Corktree bark 136, 157, 165, 180
Corn stigma 89
Corneal ulcer 144
Coronary artery 35, 46, 78
Coronary heart disease 12, 154
Cortisone 117
Corydalis tuber 85, 89, 92, 93, 130, 178
Cotinus twigs 86
Costas root 128, 150, 167

Cough 77, 85, 87, 121, 127
Crab 98
Cramps 116
Crocus sativae 168
Crohn's disease 145
Croton seed 91
Crown 108
Cucumber 98, 179
Cupping 166
Curcuma root 89, 92, 93
Cuttlefish bones 85, 90, 93, 94
Cyathula root 89, 93
Cyperus tuber 88, 93, 95, 151
Cystitis 65, 103, 104, 121, 200
Cysts 72, 73

Dahurian angelica root 92, 94
Dahurian rhododendron leaf 87
Dairy products 99, 100
Da Mo 110, 114
Damp heat 147
Dandelion 55, 86, 132, 144, 146, 151, 152, 154, 164, 167, 173, 178, 181, 185, 191, 193
Dan Gui Lu Hui Wan 78
Dang Gui Jing Pian 130
Dansen 12
Dangshen 92, 93
Datura flower 87
Deafness 38, 116, 119, 145, 152, 169
Deer 107
Dendrobium stem 90, 94, 142
Depression 37, 44, 73, 116, 130, 134, 145, 146, 163, 167, 170, 178, 180, 187
Dermatitis 56
Desert-living cistanche 90, 93, 95
Diabetes 12, 18, 43, 99, 112, 116, 128, 129, 146
Diaphragm 109, 120, 156
Diarrhoea 36, 38, 84, 85, 96, 103, 116, 120, 122, 124, 129, 131, 136, 143, 145, 146, 147, 150, 164
Dichroa root 86
Die Da Wan Hua You 131
Digestive problems 103, 119, 121, 128, 129, 132
Digitalis 82
Dinosaur fossils 85
Dittany bark 87, 164
Diuretic drugs 174, 176

Dizziness 116, 129, 146
Dodder seeds 38, 134, 145, 150, 162
Dogbane leaf 87
Dogwood fruit 90, 93, 94, 139, 140, 146, 151, 155, 156, 177
Dopamine 177
Double vision 172
Dried rehmannia root 87, 92, 93, 94, 129
Dried ginger 88, 92, 94, 142, 145, 175
Drynaria tuber 176
Duck egg 98
Duck meat 99, 168
Duodenal ulcer 151
Dwenka flower 91
Dyer's woad leaf 152
Dysentery 85, 98, 131, 147, 157
Dysmenorrhoea 78, 124, 130

Eagle wood 88
Ears 119, 120, 122, 123, 138, 145, 152, 168, 169
Earthworms 13, 85
Eating disorders 121
Eclipta 88, 145
Ectopic pregnancy 162
Eczema 56, 74, 75, 100, 116, 147
Eggshell 132
Eight Miraculous Channels 118
Eight Pieces of Brocade 110, 114
Eight principles 22
Elderflower stem and leaf 91
Electro-acupuncture 118
Emotional problems 129
Emperor Tea Pills 182
Emphysema 147
Encephalitis 47
Endangered species 127, 211
Endocrine system 72, 117, 123
Endometriosis 130, 161
Endorphins 23, 117
Enuresis 148
Ephedra 86, 92, 94, 128, 137, 154, 176
Ephedra root 90, 128
Epilepsy 12, 16, 17, 35, 57, 58, 102, 122, 134, 148
Epimedium 61, 90, 93, 94
Eucommia bark 90, 93, 94, 134, 140, 145, 162, 176

Eupatorium 87
Euphorbia root 91
Euryale seed 90
Eustachian tube 152
Evodia fruit 88, 93, 94
Exhaustion 149
Eyes 33, 36, 82, 119, 126, 144, 149
Eyesight 146, 149

Face 122, 166, 175, 182, 184, 190
Fallopian tubes 124, 160, 162
Fanggan Pian 128
Fatigue 38, 77, 130, 131, 155
Fennel fruit 88
Fennel root 36
Fermented soybean 128
Fertility 158
Fever 122, 128, 163, 167, 168, 169, 182
Fibroids 101, 124, 125, 191
Field thistle 88, 91, 92
Fire 119, 120, 124
Fish 98, 102, 103, 132
Fits 148, 149, 174
Five Animal Frolics 114
Five climates 33
Five elements 31
Five flavours 84
Five spice powder 100
Flattened milkvetch seed 89
Flatulence 149
Flavescent sophora root 86
Fleece-flower root 90, 93, 94, 138, 149, 168, 178
Fleece-flower stem 89, 130, 163
Flowering quince fruit 153
Floyer, Sir John 24
Fontanelle 169
Food 96
Food allergies 151
Food poisoning 97, 131, 149
Foot massage 123
Forgetfulness 150
Forsythia fruit 86, 92, 94, 128, 152, 181
Four diagnostic methods 39, 40, 41
Frankincense 89

Free and Easy Wanderer 36, 127, 130, 144, 146, 182
Fresh ginger 86, 90, 97, 99, 100, 102, 128, 141, 147, 150
Fritillary bulb 87, 92, 140, 179, 184
Frozen shoulder 112, 150
Fruit 96, 97, 124
Fu Ke Shi Wei Pian 130
Fu-ling 91
Fu organs 30, 120
Fu Qing-zhu 203
Fu Qing-zhu's Obstetrics and Gynaecology 203
Fu Qing-zhu's Work on Women's Diseases 203
Fu-shen 89
Futokadsura stem 91
Fu-zheng 15

Gallbladder 33, 50, 68, 69, 76, 94, 117, 120, 121, 122, 145, 150, 151, 152, 154, 155, 165, 170, 175, 183, 184
Gallstones 10, 11, 150, 165
Gangrene 69, 181
Gardenia fruit 140, 155, 157, 165
Garlic 101
Gastric disorders 121
Gastric ulcer 151
Gastroenteritis 43
Gastrodia tuber 89, 93, 147, 168, 178
Geckos 85, 128
Ge Hong 200
Ge jie lizard 12
Ge jie Dingchuan Wan 128
Genital herpes 151
Genkwa flower 87, 92, 95
Gentian root 69, 86, 93, 94
Geranium 91
Geriatric conditions 129
Germinated barley 88, 93
Germinated millet 88
Germinated rice 88
Giant hyssop 138
Giant knot weed rhizome 86
Ginger 35, 38, 97, 98, 102, 103, 142, 143, 151, 154, 156, 169, 170
Ginger stew 103
Ginger tea 171
Ginko seed 87, 90

Ginseng 38, 55, 79, 84, 90, 92, 93, 98, 129, 132, 136, 139, 141, 144, 154, 157, 162, 165, 169, 170, 173, 175, 187
Girdle channel 118
Giupi Wan 129
Glandular fever 151, 167
Glaucoma 152
Glehnia root 90, 92, 94
Glue ear 152
Glorybower leaf 89
Glossy privet fruit 90
Gold 183
Golden Lock Tea 131, 140, 158
Golden Mirror of Medicine, The 25
Golden thread 86, 146, 147
Gout 153
Governor vessel 102, 117, 118, 121, 122
Grains of paradise 149
Granula anularis 58
Grass-leaved sweet-flag rhizome 89, 92, 94
Grassy privet 146, 156
Great envelope of the spleen 118
Great Herbal 34, 78, 82, 196, 201
Great Ormond Street Children's Hospital 74
Green chiretta 86
Green tangerine peel 88
Groin 151, 152, 189
Grommet 152
Growth problems 38
Guillian Barre syndrome 59, 153
Guy, Dr Geoffrey 74
Gwenka flower 92, 93
Gynaecological complaints 82, 101, 123, 124, 125, 126 130
Gypsum 86, 92, 94, 163, 169, 178, 191

Haematite 89
Haemorrhoids 116, 153
Hair 32, 138
Hale-White, William 81
Handbook of Prescriptions for Emergencies 200
Hawthorn fruit 88, 93, 94, 137, 140, 158
Hay fever 36, 60, 116, 154, 184
Head 108, 121, 168, 175
Headache 105, 116, 120, 128, 154, 163, 168, 170

Heart 30, 31, 32, 33, 34, 50, 75, 84, 92, 99, 108, 117, 119, 121, 124, 135, 139, 148, 155, 177, 185
Heart attack 13, 155
Heartbeat 111, 177
Heartburn 132, 156
Heavenly qi 119
Hedysarum root 90
Hemlock 82
Hemp seed 87, 94, 95
Henbane seed 87
Hen's eggs 98, 100, 102
Hepatitis 77, 116, 155, 192
Herbal tea 144, 145, 178
Hernia 122
Herpes 37, 116
Hiatus hernia 156
Hiccups 156
HIV 76, 79, 133
Hives 174
Hodgkin's disease 156
Honey 84, 86
Honeylocust thorn 88
Honeysuckle 69, 86, 129, 142, 144, 152, 163, 178
Honeysuckle flower 86, 92, 94, 95, 105, 128, 140, 165, 168, 173, 175, 182
Hormone imbalance 175
Hormone replacement therapy 123
Hot flushes 130, 170
Houttuynia 86, 179
Hsing yi 114
Huangfu-Mi 200
Huang Kuan 27
Huangqi 78
Hua Tuo 24, 76, 106, 114
Hu Si-hui 96, 202
Hunan province 110
Huo Xiang Zheng Qi Yuan 131
Hyacinth bletilla 88, 92, 93, 94
Hypertension 112
Hyperventilation 136
Hypoglycaemia 116
Hypoglauca yam 91
Hypothalamus 117
Hystermyoma 124

Ileum 145
Immature bitter oranges 88, 93, 94, 95
Immune system 38, 49, 77, 78, 133, 141, 156, 168
Imperata rhizome 87, 89
Impetigo 157
Impotence 84, 116, 157
Incontinence 121, 131, 140, 158
Indian chrysanthemum flower 86
Indigestion 116, 128, 144, 149, 158
Indigo 152
Infertility 37, 61, 116, 119, 158, 177
Influenza 22, 35, 52, 78, 97, 116, 117, 128, 129, 146, 163, 174
Intestines 138, 147, 164
Irregular periods 116, 130
Insomnia 116, 122, 124, 129, 130, 163, 164
Institute of Materia Medica, Beijing 76, 78, 83
Insulin 18, 146
Inula flower 87, 92, 93, 94, 95
Iris pallasi seeds 78
Irisquinone 78
Irritable bowel syndrome 164
Itching 164
Isatis leaf 69, 86, 92, 94
Isatis root 86 92, 173
I-Yin 96,

Japanese dioscorea rhizome 91
Japanese fern spores 91
Japanese thistle 89, 153
Jaundice 76, 77, 85, 155, 164
Jaw 122
Jia, Professor Hing Han 117
Jing 86, 108, 113, 133, 159
Jinglao 117
Jin Hi Chongji 130
Jin Suo Gu Jing Wan 131
Junction channels 118
Jung Chang 113

Kansui root 91, 92, 93, 95
Kapok flower 141, 146, 154
Katsumadai seed 87
Key to the Therapeutics of Children's Diseases 201

Kidneys 30, 31, 32, 35, 37, 50, 55, 68, 72, 84, 85, 91, 93, 108, 117, 119, 120, 121, 122, 123, 124, 126, 128, 129, 130, 131, 133, 134, 137, 138, 139, 140, 142, 144, 145, 146, 148, 150, 152, 153, 156, 157, 158, 159, 160, 162, 163,164, 168, 169, 170, 171, 172, 173, 174, 175, 176, 177, 178 182, 185, 186, 190, 193
Kidney stones 153
Knees 128
Knoxia root 87, 92, 93, 95
Korean ginseng 149
Kudzu vine 90, 134

Lamb 101, 102
Laminaria 87
Large intestine 50, 95, 117, 120, 121, 120
Large-leaf gentian root 91, 136
Lao Tzu 109, 195
Laryngitis 131, 165
Lateral root of aconite 88, 92, 93, 94
Leafy vegetables 98
Ledebouriella root 86, 90, 93, 94, 147, 174, 176
Leg ulcers 62
Lemongrass 87
Lens 144, 152
Lepidium seed 87, 92, 94, 179
Leucorrhoea 130, 131
Leukaemia 77, 78, 164
Li Gao 201
Liang Dynasty 114
Lichen planus 165
Ligament problems 119, 166
Light wheat 90, 92
Ligustrum lucidum 15, 78
Lily bulb 87, 90, 92, 99
Lily root 172, 173
Lilyturf root 36, 90, 140, 146, 155, 177, 181, 186
Limonite 85
Ling Shu 196
Liquorice 38, 77, 90, 92, 93, 94, 97, 128, 132, 139, 146, 151, 155, 156
Li Shi zhen 25, 78, 82, 202
Liu Jun Zi Wan 129
Liver 15, 30, 31, 32, 33, 34, 36, 37, 38, 39, 50, 68, 73, 75, 76, 77, 79, 84, 89, 91, 92, 102, 103, 117, 119, 120, 121, 122, 124, 125, 126, 128, 130, 132, 134, 136, 137, 138, 139, 140, 142, 144,145, 146, 149, 150, 151, 152, 153, 154, 155, 156,
, 160, 162, 163, 164, 165, 167, 170, 171, 175, 176, 177, 178, 179, 180, 182, 184, 185, 186, 187, 190, 191, 192, 193

Liver meridian 102, 124
Lobster 98
Loganberry fruit 136
Long pepper 88
Lophatherum 86, 128
Loquat leaf 87
Loranthus 87
Loranthus mulberry mistletoe 87, 93
Lotus node 88
Lotus seeds 35, 90, 93, 94
Lotus stamen 90
Lovage tuber 154, 178, 186
Low sperm count 6, 128, 131, 162, 185
Lucid ganoderma 89
Lui Wei Di Huang Wan 128, 131
Lulu Daoyin 115
Lumbago 122, 128, 131, 166
Lungs 30, 31, 32, 33, 34, 35, 36, 37, 45, 51, 67, 68, 75, 84, 91, 92, 117, 119, 120, 121, 122, 123, 128, 137, 140, 146, 147, 148, 154, 155, 165, 174, 175, 176, 179, 184
Luo, Dr Ding Hui 74
Lupus (systemic lupus erythematosus) 56, 166
Lu Tzu 115
Lymphoma 69
Lymph glands 78, 151, 152, 156
Lysimachia 87, 91, 92, 94, 151
Lystena 149

Macrophage cells 79, 133
Macrostem onion 88, 92, 94, 95, 135
Madder root 167
Magnolia bark 88, 92, 95, 141, 144, 149, 151, 154, 156, 164
Magnolia flower 86, 142, 154
Mai Jing 45, 198
Mafeisan 198
Malaria 76, 78, 122, 166, 171
Malt extract 90
Manchurian aristolochia stem 91, 92, 94, 95
Manchurian lilac bark 87
Manic depression 119
Manipulation 46, 138, 166
Mastitis 104, 167
Mao Zedong 27, 203
Massage 138, 143, 150, 163, 166
Mawangdui 110

ME 47, 62, 63, 70, 167, 168
Measles 168
Meat 96. 97, 99, 100, 101, 168, 186
Meniere's disease 169
Meningitis 35, 134,169
Menopause 53, 73, 124, 130, 170
Menstrual cycle 101, 113, 121, 177
Menstrual problems 42, 119, 122, 123, 129, 130, 158, 169
Meridians 23, 30, 91, 107, 108, 118, 122, 138
Metabolism 175, 178, 189, 193
Miscarriage 102, 123, 162, 171
Migraine 112, 122, 125, 130, 154, 162, 170
Milk 57, 103, 132
Minor burns 104
Millettia stem 166
Mirabilite 94, 95
Mistletoe 38, 65
Morinda root 38
Morning sickness 102, 171
Mosquito bites 104, 166, 171
Mother-of-pearl 89
Motherwort 89, 92, 93, 94
Motor neurone disease 63, 64
Moutan bark 92, 93
Mouth ulcers 35, 70, 171
Moxibustion 116, 123, 153, 163, 170, 172, 177, 188
Mugwort 172
Mulberry bark 87, 157
Mulberry fruit 134, 138, 139, 145, 146, 147, 149, 150, 156, 190
Mulberry leaf 36, 38, 86, 92, 93, 140, 154, 165, 175, 182, 196
Mulberry-leafed chrysanthemum 90
Mulberry mistletoe 65, 86
Mulberry twigs 176, 188
Multiple sclerosis 65, 66, 172
Mumps 173
Muscles 114, 119
Muscular dystrophy 67, 173
Mustard seed 101
Mutton 99, 102
Myalgic encephalomyelitis see ME
Myelin sheath 172
Myocarditis 13, 173
Myrrh 89

Nanjing 66
National Association for Chinese Medicine 27
National Eczema Society 74
Nausea 36, 77, 97, 129, 135, 136, 139, 150, 154, 155, 167, 168, 169, 170, 174
Neck 109, 111, 116, 122, 135, 143, 152, 156, 166, 169, 189, 190
Nei dan 107, 114
Nei Jing 21, 31, 45, 96, 107, 110, 112, 159, 195, 196, 200
Nephritis 36, 174
Nettle rash 174
Nervous problems 122, 155
Nervous system 157, 163, 172
Neuralgia 116, 122, 175
Neurodermatitis 85
Night sweats 130
Niuhuang Yijin Pian 131
Non-specific urethritis 162
Nose and throat 119, 175
Nosebleeds 60, 117
Notoginseng 88, 93, 94, 151, 166, 178
Notopterygium root 91, 94
Nu Bao 130
Nutgrass flatsedge rhizome 130
Nutmeg 90

Obesity 38, 99, 175
Obsessional behaviour 44
Oedema 29, 36, 38, 46, 174, 175, 179
Oesophagus 156
Oldenlandia black nightshade 86
'Old Man's Eyebrows' 100
Omphalia 88
Ophiopogon root 92, 94, 129
Optic nerve 152, 184
Optic neuritis 66, 67
Orange peel 132, 137, 141, 142, 149, 156, 169, 180
Oriental water plantain rhizome 87, 93, 94
Oriental wormwood 87, 93, 94, 138, 147, 155, 165
Osteoarthritis 136, 176,
Osteoporosis 66, 170, 176
Ovaries 124, 125, 159, 160, 173
Ovulation problems 177
Oyster shells 85, 89, 193

Pagoda-tree flower 88

Palm oil 104, 171
Palpitations 73, 122, 129, 136, 155, 177, 189
Pancreas 38, 146, 150
Panic attacks 136
Paniculate swallow-wort root 91
Pao Po Tzu 110
Paralysis 122, 153, 179, 186, 2000
Paris rhizome 86
Parkinson's disease 29, 97, 177
Patent medicines 127
Patient rumex root 88
Patrinia herb 86
Peach kernel 62, 89, 92, 93, 95, 136
Peanuts 97, 103
Pears 104, 128
Peking spurge root 91
Pelvic inflammatory disease 116, 123, 130
Peony 104, 132, 144, 152, 186, 192
Peony bark 167, 178
Peony buds 178
Peony root 37, 38, 97, 130, 137, 139, 147, 156, 170, 175, 185
Peppercorns 104
Peppermint 86, 92, 93, 128, 138, 142, 145, 146, 163, 165, 168, 175, 183, 184
Peptic ulcer 128, 178
Pericardium 34, 50, 95, 117, 120, 121, 122
Perilla leaf 86, 90
Perilla seed 87, 92, 95
Perilla stem 149, 156
Perineum 108, 118, 121
Peuraria root 129
Pharbitis seed 91
Pharyngitis 131
Pheasant 101
Phellodendron bark 86, 94, 95, 131
Phlebitis 178
Phlegm 129, 137, 179, 193
Phytolacca root 91
Pigeon pea 152
Pig's tail 98
Piles 153
Pilose asiabell root 90, 128
Pimples 104, 178
Pinellia tuber 87, 92, 93, 94, 128, 141
Pink 91

Pink eye 179
Plantain 91, 104, 151, 152, 180
Plantain seed 87, 92, 93, 140, 145, 151, 175
Plastron 85
Platycodon root 87, 92, 128, 129
PMT 37, 116, 124, 130, 160, 161, 179
Pneumonia 51, 179
Poliomyelitis 116, 179
Polished rice 100
Polygala root 89, 92
Pomegranate 105
Pomegranate rind 90
Pomelo peel 88
Poppy capsule 90
Poppy heads 87
Poria 87, 92, 93, 94, 128, 132, 141, 144, 145, 154, 163, 164, 170, 175, 180
Pork 99, 101, 102, 103
Prawns 98
Pregnancy 45, 51, 102, 135, 144, 150, 159, 162, 179, 182, 192
Prickly-ash peel 88
Prostate 68, 158, 180
Prunella spike 87
Pseudostellaria root 90
Psoralea fruit 90, 93, 94, 146
Psoriasis 56, 68, 69, 85, 180
Pubescent angelica root 87, 91, 93, 94, 136, 176
Pubescent holly root 89
Pueraria root 86, 90, 93
Puffball 87
Pulsatilla root 87, 95
Pulse diagnosis 22, 39, 40, 45, 50, 200
Pulses (food) 99, 101
Pumpkin seed 88, 94, 95
Puncture vine fruit 164
Purple cowrie shells 89
Purple perilla 90
Purslane 86
Pyrrosia leaf 91, 151

Qi 13, 18, 22, 23, 30, 106, 107, 108, 109, 110, 111, 112, 114, 115, 118, 119, 121, 129, 130, 131, 139, 145, 155, 156, 166, 168, 169, 170, 172, 176, 177, 180
Qi gong 18, 19, 46, 106, 107, 108, 109, 110, 111, 112, 113, 114
Qian Yi 201
Qi Ju Di Huang Wan 130

Qinghao 76
Quinine 167
Quinsy 181
Quisqualis fruit 88, 93, 94

Radical lobelia 86
Radiotherapy 141, 156
Radish seed 88, 92, 93, 94, 136, 138
Raspberry 90
Raynaud's disease 69, 181
Red halloysite 85
Red meat 98
Red ochre 85
Red peony root 86, 89, 92, 130, 135, 152
Red sage 13, 35, 89, 92, 95, 135, 137, 142, 155
Reed rhizome 87
Rehmannia root 61, 130, 141, 172, 173
Renal artery 78
Restlessness 129, 130, 163, 181
Return Spleen Tablets 129, 133, 134, 169, 174
Rhinoceros horn 164, 211
Rhubarb 55, 87, 93, 95, 104, 132, 143, 144, 145, 151, 152, 154, 156, 164, 167, 172, 173, 175, 178, 182, 185, 187, 191
Rheumatism 85, 181, 182, 200, 211
Rheumatoid arthritis 66, 67, 70, 71, 104, 136, 182
Ribcage 109
Rice sprouts 136, 140, 158
Root vegetables 98
Round cardamom seed 87
Royal Free Hospital, London 16, 69, 103
Royal jelly 149
Rubella 182
Rubia root 88
Rush pith 91
Safflower 62, 70, 89, 92, 93, 135, 165
Saffron 89, 137, 142, 178
Sage 139
Saliva glands 173
Salmonella 149
Sanguisorba root 88, 93, 94, 95
Sanjiao 117
Sappan wood 89
Sargassum seaweed 87
Scandent hops 86

Schisandra fruit 90
Schizonepeta 90, 92, 93, 128, 147, 174, 182
Schizophrenia 17, 35, 122, 163, 182
Sciatica 116, 121, 131, 138, 183
Scleroderma 69
Scorpions 85
Scrofula 85
Scrophularia root 69, 87, 90, 92, 94
Scutellaria root 65, 92, 94, 95
Sea-ear shell 89
Seahorse 85, 157
Seasickness 183
Seaweed 97, 190, 211
Self-heal scutellarea root 86, 144, 145
Semen 61, 113, 159
Senna leaf 87
Sesame oil 104, 132, 144, 182, 192
Sesame seeds 103, 144
Seven-lobed yam 91
Sexual dysfunction 120
Sextone 140, 157, 169
Shang Shi Zhi Ton Gao 131
Shang Han Za Bing Lun 198
Shaolin temple 110, 114
Shave grass 86
Shen 17, 34, 108, 163, 182
Shen Nung 82
Shepherd's purse 88
Shingles 46, 183, 184
Shoulder 122, 150
Shu points 122
Siberian solomonseal rhizome 90
Sichuan aconite root, 88
Sichuan clematis stem 91
Siegesbeckia herb 91
Silken tofu 103
Silk vine bark 91
Sinus problems 116, 119, 184
Six Gentlemen 127, 129, 140, 148, 173
Six Noble Ingredients 128
Six Healing Sounds 114
Six Rehmannia Pills 128, 130, 131, 172, 174
Sjogren's Syndrome 69
Skeletal problems 119, 121

Skin problems 102, 120
Skullcap root 36, 86, 140, 145, 146, 147, 151, 152, 154, 157, 170, 173, 175, 178
Slipped disc 72, 166, 183, 184
Small intestine 33, 38, 43, 50, 95, 117, 120, 121, 122, 186
Small thistle 88
Smilax China-root 25
Smilax glabra rhizome 86
Snake 85
Snakebed seed 86
Snake gourd root 79, 87, 133, 167
Snake skin 164
Spastic colon 164, 185
Sore throat 85, 116
Spatholobus stem 89, 130
Speech impediment 119
Sperm count 128, 131, 158, 160, 161
Sperm disorders 185
Spirodela 86, 92
Spine 98, 107, 136, 173, 176, 183, 184
Spleen 30, 31, 32, 33, 34, 35, 36, 38, 42, 50. 73, 84, 91, 93, 101, 103, 117, 118, 119, 121, 122, 123, 124, 129, 132, 133, 134, 135, 136, 137, 138, 139, 140, 143, 144, 145, 146, 149, 156, 158, 160, 164, 169, 170, 171, 172, 173, 174, 175, 178, 180, 185, 186, 187, 190, 191, 193
Sports injuries 131
Spots 178, 185
Sprains 116
Spring and Autumn Annals 115
Spring onion tea 97, 105, 154
Squid bone 178
Staphylococcus 149
Stellaria root 87
Stemona root 87
Sterility 130, 173
Stomach 30, 33, 36, 37, 38, 42, 43, 50, 77, 94, 97, 101, 103, 112, 117, 121, 122, 131, 132, 132, 134, 138, 140, 143, 144, 145, 146, 147, 149, 150, 151, 152, 154, 156, 158, 163, 164, 168, 170, 171, 172, 173, 174, 178, 185, 191, 193
Stomach pains 147
Stomach ulcers 77, 112
Storax 89
Stress 116, 119, 136, 137, 145, 151, 155, 159, 165, 167, 168, 174, 183, 187
Stroke 16, 29, 77, 116, 154, 185
Subprostrate sophora root 86
Sun Si Miao 114
Sweating 125, 128, 131, 163, 186, 189

Sweet flag root 149
Sweetgum fruit 91
Sweet wormwood 87, 92, 93, 94, 101
Swallow-wort root 87
Swollen glands 162, 173
Tachycardia 177
Tai qi 19, 107, 114, 176
Tao 108, 194-195
Tao Hong Jing 200
Taoism 109, 194-195, 200
Tamarisk tops 86
Tangerine peel 38, 62, 88, 92, 93, 103, 128, 184
Tangerine seed 88
Tan-Kuei 102
Tan T'ien 108
Tapeworms 186
Tartarian aster root 128
TATT (Tired All The Time syndrome) 187
T-cells 77, 78, 79, 133
Tea 97, 100, 103, 104
Teasel root 138
Teeth 122, 187
Tendon disorders 116, 187
Tendrilled fritillary bulb 87
Testicles 159, 160, 173, 185
Tetrandra root 87, 91, 93, 94
Thistle 174, 175
Thorowax root 37, 86, 136, 145, 146, 154, 156, 170, 180, 185
Threadworms 188
Three Treasures 108
Thrush 189
Thrusting channel 118
Throat 116, 119, 122, 128, 131, 165, 174, 175, 181, 190
Thunberg fritillary bulb 87
Thyroid 72, 84, 177, 189
Tianjin First Teaching Hospital 10, 12, 13, 15, 16, 17, 18, 40, 56, 78, 85, 124, 147, 155
Tian Wang Bu Xin Dan 129
Tic 190
Timos-pora stem 176
Tinnitus 38, 116, 119, 122, 128, 130, 145, 190
Toad venom 85
Tongue 22, 33, 34, 35, 41, 42, 47, 53, 63
Tonics 90, 91, 99, 100, 102, 103, 139
Tonsillitis 35, 105, 131, 152, 162, 174, 181, 190

Toothache 82, 191
Torrya seed 88
Travel sickness 191
Treatise on Febrile Diseases 198
Tree of heaven bark 86
Tree peony bark 47
Tribulus fruit 89
Trichosanthes fruit 87, 92, 94
Trichosanthin 76, 79, 133
Triple burner 30, 117, 120, 121, 122
Tripterytium wilfordii 182
Trophoblast cells 79, 133
Tsaoko 87
Tuberculosis 112
Tumour 78, 85, 112, 117
Turmeric 89, 150
Turtle 128
Typhonium tuber 87

Ulcers 85, 116, 122, 151
Ulcerated colitis 191
Umbellate pore-fungus 91, 94
Uncaria stem 89, 93, 95
Uric acid 153
Urine 139, 148
Urticaria 174
Uterine disorders 162, 191
Uterine polyps 125
Uterus 38, 101, 102, 124, 125, 131, 191

Vaccaria seeds 89
Vagina 151
Vaginitis 116
Valerian rhizome 89
Varicose ulcers 192
Varicose veins 192
Vegetable sponge 91
Venison 101
Vervain 89
Vertigo 130, 192
Viola herb 86
Violet 132, 179
Viral meningitis 169
Virus infections 155, 192

Vomiting 77, 84, 124, 140, 150, 168, 169, 174

Walnuts 98, 148
Wang Ang 203
Wang Anshi 26
Wang bu liu xing zi 123
Wang Xi 198
Warts 193
Wasps' nests 85
Water 33, 98, 100, 119, 120, 124, 147
Watermelon 104, 134, 179
Water plantain 139, 146, 151, 174, 180
Wei 22
Wei dan 107, 114
Weight problems 193
Wheat 98
Wheat sprouts 136, 140, 157
White atractylodes rhizome 90, 93, 94, 176
White mustard seed 87, 92
White peony root 90, 92, 93, 136, 146, 147, 178, 180, 185
White tiger decoction 169
Wild aconite root 88
Wild angelica 139, 154
Wild boar 101
Wild chrysanthemum 132, 179
Wild game 101
Wild ginger 86, 136, 154
Wild jujube seed 89, 92, 93, 154, 163, 177
Wintercherry fruit 86
Wolfberry bark 86, 92, 94, 185
Wolfberry fruit 90, 92, 93, 94, 137, 138, 142, 147, 149, 157, 165, 168
Wolfberry root 141
Wolfberry seed 134
Women's Precious Pills 125, 127, 130, 177, 191
Worms 104
Wu Ji Bai Feng Wan 130
Wu Youxing 203

Xanthium fruit 86, 184
Xiao Yan Wan 130
Xue 22

Yang qi 109, 142, 155
Yanlixiao Jiaonang 131

Yan Xiao-zhong 201
Yellow Emperor 96, 110, 159
Ye Tian Si 22
Yeuh Fei 110, 114
Yin-yang concept 27, 29, 50, 52, 61, 78, 80, 84, 97, 98, 118, 120, 126, 141, 185
Yin Qiao Jie Du Pian 128
Yin qiao mo 118
Yin wei mo 118
Ying 22
Yeuh-chukene 77
Yun zhi 77

Zang organs 30, 120
Zemaphyte 75
Zhang Cong-zhen 201
Zhang-Lu 203
Zhang Zhong-jing 26, 99
Zhe Bai Di Huang Wan 130
Zhisou Dingchuan Gao 128
Zhong qi 101
Zodoary 89
Zhu Zhen-heng 201

Printed in Great Britain
by Amazon